YOUR GREATEST WEALTH

9 Steps to Optimizing Your Health and Happiness

TONY BE

Dedication

I dedicate this book to the health
and evolution of humanity

Table of Contents

Acknowledgements

I ACKNOWLEDGE THE SUPPORT AND love from my parents. I thank my Yogi family all around the world for showing me what kindness really is and for that quality of seeing the best in me. I am thankful to all the nutritional teachers from whom I have learnt. I thank my friend Andy Morey for sharing his extensive knowledge in natural healing and I acknowledge all the healing sessions I have received that have shown me new insights into my own healing. I thank Raymond Arron who motivated me to write this book, and the team from Automated Business System who have helped me incorporate everything I have learnt into a way I can truly make a living out of doing something I love, which benefits so many people around the world. I thank Andy Harrington for teaching me public speaking. There have been so many teachers in my life, literally; so I thank you all for what you have shared with me.

Foreword

ARE YOU LOOKING FOR HEALTHIER options in your life? However, it is not as simple as it sounds to change your lifestyle. It is necessary to acquire the right knowledge and enhance your awareness of the relationships between lifestyle and health.

Where can you find the right factors, suggestions, or methods to increase your health in order to get that healthy lifestyle? You have all the answers you need for a healthier lifestyle in your hands.

Antony Be has studied natural health care for more than 20 years. He discovered a general natural health system that could literally help you improve your overall health. All his secrets are revealed to you within this book, Your Greatest Wealth.

Disease and ill-health do not only occur by chance as the majority of chronic or longstanding diseases, they are often related to unhealthy lifestyle habits—for example, smoking, a bad diet, physical inactivity and the list could go on and on. These conditions are known as lifestyle diseases and many of the determinants of health are well known.

Antony's system consists of 9 steps to increase your overall health in order to add the best healthy elements to your life by improving your health and happiness. The content in this book is a truly amazing testimony of beating cancer. Antony shares his own experience that is easy to follow. This book is practical, honest and fresh of ideas to encourage you to start living and embracing life.

Your Greatest Wealth is your health; this book has the potential to make a huge positive difference in your life.

So get ready to read these incredible insights to your greatest wealth.

Raymond Aaron
New York Times Best Selling Author

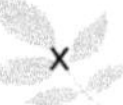

x

Introduction

IN 1988, AT THE AGE of fourteen, I was diagnosed with ulcerative colitis and in 2010, aged thirty-five, diagnosed with cancer of the large intestine. In my early teens, despite all the conventional treatment, I was still having really tough symptoms. This led me from an early age to study and to learn anything that could help me reduce my symptoms.

I've studied natural health care intensively for over twenty years. In doing so, I've discovered a general natural health system that could help literally anyone improve their overall health or help prevent an illness in the first place.

This book is for people who wish to get healthy and stay healthy. It's also for people who would like to reduce the symptoms of an autoimmune disease such as ulcerative colitis/crohns disease, or are recovering from chronic illness and looking for natural health protocols to help stay healthy.

This book and online training course have grown out of what I have learnt over the years, and I wish I had known this stuff 20 years ago.

Because I know what it is like to suffer, physically and mentally, from a long term illness, I also know the feeling of relief that comes when you start making improvements. It is this good stuff that I'll share with you here.

THIS HAS NEVER BEEN MORE URGENT

If you're willing to join me on this journey to discover Your Greatest Wealth, we need first to pull back the veil and see what is really going on in society, because I believe we're sitting on a health time bomb for the next generation. Let me explain why.

A 2011/12 survey from the UK reported that 65% of men and 58% of women in England are classed as either overweight or obese, 1 in 2 people are dying of heart disease and 1 in 2 are diagnosed with cancer. Breast cancer has increased from 1 in 20 in 1968 to 1 in 7 today. One tenth of children aged between four and five are classed as obese. Some newborn babies are born with over two hundred industrial chemicals in their bodies. One in two children has a chronic illness such as asthma, autism, autoimmune disease or diabetes. In 1980, 1 in 2000 children had Autism, and today it's 1 in 150 the CDC estimates. It is now predicted that children today are expected to live ten years less than their parents: this is the first time in history that such a dramatic decrease in lifespan between adjacent generations has been forecast.

So even though this current generation is living longer than ever before and everything looks as though health issues are improving, underneath the fact is that there is something going seriously wrong and many people are simply turning a blind eye to it.

Sadly, until they lose their health, too many people take it for granted. Often when their health fails they rely on their doctor to fix them, which is all well and good, but people seem to be losing general common sense in terms of caring for their own health.

THE BEST OF BOTH WORLDS

Sure, you can eat all the junk you want… here's a pill for high blood pressure. Don't exercise at all… here's a pill for obesity. That stress is no biggie… here's a pill to alter your mood. Gobble up excessive sugar… we have your insulin ready.

The downside is that people are still looking for that quick fix and don't want to take responsibility for their own basic health. Where have we lost our way, treating symptoms on such a huge scale without really looking at the underlying cause? And yes there is a huge amount of confusion out there, with one science paper saying this, and another paper saying something else, and this natural practitioner saying one thing and another saying the opposite. Over the years, my approach has been to listen, then use common logic, then test it out, and then see the results.

The World Health Organization acknowledges that between 70-85% of all disease is caused by what we put into our mouths and by lack of physical movement. Yet the stumbling block lies in people's mindset. Generally, people have a knee-jerk reaction to basic nutritional advice, natural remedies or therapies, saying, "That can't be any good if it is not mainstream," or, "if it was any good it would be mainstream."

The confusing issue is that it makes no sense for the large pharmaceuticals to spend a lot of money on research into what prevents an illness. Their job (and their business) is treating illness with a drug they can make a profit on, either by successfully treating a condition in a short period or managing the symptoms. I see a place for pharmaceutical drug companies, as their drugs have literally saved my life and helped me have surgeries with very little pain. However, I believe we do need to look elsewhere for prevention and, for generally looking after ourselves on a daily basis, to give ourselves the best of both worlds.

Dr. M. Grey, one of Britain's most senior doctors and the chief knowledge officer for the NHS, said, "The overuse of medication is one of the most serious problems we face today."

There are more antibiotic-resistant bacteria being discovered as people, in a pill-popping frenzy, continue to overuse their doctors to get that quick-fix prescription. I believe if we are not clever enough as a human race and keep abusing pharmaceutical drugs instead of dealing with the basics of keeping ourselves healthy, we are heading for Pharma-Armageddon. This is going beyond germ theory of Louis Pasteur in 1861, because gems are everywhere, it is about our terrain, our internal and external environment, how strong our cells are. What are your beliefs about health and happiness in your life?

It's my belief that we need the best of both worlds. Because people are suffering needlessly around the world, if we can combine the best knowledge of mainstream medicine with the best of integrated medicine (what people can do for themselves in their daily life to strengthen their health and wellbeing), we're onto a winning formula.

DEVELOPING HEALTHY HABITS

People are becoming more aware that if you have habitual healthy lifestyle habits you are likely to live at least an extra 10–20 years, and enjoy your life even more. It is pretty much common sense when you think about it for a moment but the question is, what are those healthy habits?

On my own health journey, what I noticed was that I got one or two areas of healthy living right in my life but, because I didn't yet understand how the other areas came together, I was only getting OK results. As soon as I worked out how these areas fitted together, I told myself I was finally ready to share this with the world.

I use to practice a lot of martial arts. The skills of a great MMA fighter combine different arts such as grappling, judo throws, punches, kicks and arts like aikido where you work with the life force, or chi. But if you just practice judo in that arena you will not have the support of those other skills. I see the same thing with natural health care: we need to combine different elements together to create a great healing system.

From this insight I've created for my clients the Greatest Wealth Generator which is the pie chart below. This book will show you the easy, effective steps that will enable you to personalise and integrate these insights into your daily life, plus I have also created an online video course that will help you even further understand and implement all these 9 steps.

Each chapter could easily be a whole book. What you'll find here is some of the best of the best information from each of these sections, so you can really get to see for yourself how they all work together. This is the overview map of this book:

YOUR GREATEST WEALTH HEALTH GENERATOR

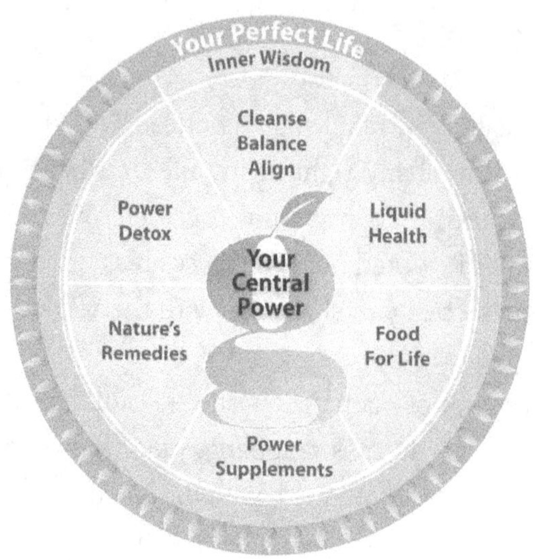

To summarise each step:

1. *"Cleanse, Balance, Align"* looks at how many people unknowingly and unnecessarily slightly poison themselves on a daily basis and suggests which foods and environmental factors are best avoided. You will find out about the consequences of a depletion of minerals, vitamins and essential oils in your life and how to rebalance them; also how to ease and reduce back pain.

2. *"Liquid Health"* is about how to create your own tonic bar. You will soon realize that one of the easiest ways to improve your health is to simply drink more healthy drinks! You'll learn how to make some of the healthiest and most tasty drinks you've ever tried.

3. *"Food for Life"* doesn't push more restricted diets, but describes how to create an awesome personal food plan based on 9 food factors, which I'll introduce.

4. *"Power Supplements"* is your chance to discover the key health supplements that can benefit your body and help you perform at your optimum in all areas of your life.

5. *"Nature's Remedies"* reveals five natural remedies for a better quality of life—from getting the best night's sleep to improving your joints, treating a common cold or improving your skin tone.

6. *"Power Detox"* shows you two intensive detoxes: one to help clear Candida fungus, and the second to achieve a successful liver and gallbladder flush.

7. *"Inner Wisdom"* introduces an inner space of clarity and calm that each of us has. I show you how you can rest in this space on a daily basis, often resulting in a happier life.

8. *"Power of You"*—this chapter shows how when you've been ill you can unknowingly play the victim and diminish your power. You will learn how to pull back your power and remain centred, whatever is happening in your life.

9. *"Your Perfect Life"* is about setting goals. Whether you have a health goal, a dream to go to Disney, or a goal to turn your passion into your work, living your dreams has a huge effect on your health and your mindset. In this chapter you will learn insights and techniques which will inspire you to live your dreams.

This is a brief overview. As you'll soon see, there is much more to be found.

About the Author

ANTONY'S NICKNAME IS TONY BE and his parents owned a small corner shop selling everything from handbags to grandfather clocks in Torbay, Devon. They started with a very small loan and built up a large luggage importing company from almost nothing. Both his parents worked really hard, so much so that Tony would hardly see them when he was growing up.

At fourteen he was at a boys' boarding school in Bournemouth, where he got bullied; at the same time his parents were getting divorced.

The hardest part for him at that stage of his life was that he felt all alone and didn't know who to turn to. As he didn't know how to deal with all his emotions, they got bottled up inside him. He was diagnosed with ulcerative colitis, which is ulceration of the large intestine—a condition they say cannot be cured although it can be managed.

The doctors put him on large amounts of steroids and immuno-suppressants, which worked for some of the time, but came with unpleasant side effects.

Over the years he managed the symptoms and lived what looked like a normal working life from the outside, yet it was really challenging for him. By the age of 18 he was running wholesale luggage warehouses in Birmingham and the East End of London, dealing with highly stressful situations, which resulted in more flare-ups of ulcerative colitis.

So, from an early age, Tony started getting really interested in what could help. Food seemed an obvious place to start so, alongside his main job, he did a part-time one-year course in Food Energetics and Nutrition with the International Macrobiotic School in Bath.

Then, as he was getting some Shiatsu massages, he developed a fascination with how Chinese medicine worked and took a three-year diploma course in Shiatsu Massage.

He found that Yoga and Mediation also helped a lot, so he also studied for three years part time on a Dru Yoga Teacher training course.

Even though he knew all of this information and practised these powerful healing techniques, he was still having major health issues.

So at 32 he quit his main job and moved to Portugal where he taught Yoga and gave Shiatsu Massages. Life was pretty good for him at this period, yet the ulcerative colitis was still in the background all the time.

Three years later, this turned into cancer of the large intestine. His consultant recommended he should have his whole large intestine removed.

At this point Tony had been trying to manage his symptoms for over nineteen years, going from one so-called expert to another. Mentally, he'd had enough.

So he decided to go ahead with the surgery, which was a successful operation that gave him an internal pouch made from part of his small intestine. It works really well, and he sincerely thanks the surgeon who did a really great job.

At the same time, he wishes he had known 20 years earlier what he knows now. He now believes the insights in his book and training course could have helped him get his colitis into remission and helped him avoid getting cancer in the first place, yet he also realizes he is the person he is today because of what he has been through.

Now, by combining all his experiences, training courses and personal research, he has created the Your Greatest Wealth coaching system which includes all the best of what he has learnt over the years and how all these different areas of healing work together. You're holding in your hands some of the most fundamental tips he was searching for twenty years ago.

THE GOLDEN TICKET

In life we all age and that's normal. Yet many of us suffer from auto-immune disease, heart disease, joint pain, diabetes and many other degenerative diseases because we don't take care of ourselves and our bodies. We are not properly educated about the most valuable thing we have, which is our health. Then, 'out of nowhere', people are getting cancer, heart disease etc. and they think it is just bad luck. But often it's not: it's an accumulation of factors that the nine areas of this book seek to address.

The Golden Ticket you get with this book—good health—doesn't need to be hard to achieve. I will share with you how to enjoy healthy living, not to treat it as a chore or to be extreme with it, rather to celebrate it, and enjoy it so much that it is a natural choice, and sometimes zigzag with it so sometimes you can have or do anything: have that chocolate fudge sundae sometimes, you can have anything now and then, you have that freedom. Yet once you feel this vitality you won't want to go back.

Many people are consumed in life with the question of where to invest. Should they invest in property? Or in stocks and shares? In this book you will discover your greatest investment is in your health.

You can read this book in whatever way you prefer. One suggestion is to read one chapter per week and fully implement the suggestions made in each one. You're welcome to join the online course that accompanies this book and provides deeper information into how this all works and how to make it come alive.

Healthy living starts with your mindset! So are you ready to come on the journey to truly discover Your Greatest Wealth?

"Health is like money,
we never have a true idea of
its value until we lose it!"

~ JOSH BILLINGS

Cleanse, Balance, Align

YOUR FIRST STEP TO HEALTHY living is understanding the three main causes of health issues today. By knowing and addressing each of these you can reduce the symptoms of an existing health condition or, better still, look at this as prevention rather than a cure.

"Every so-called disease is a crisis of Toxemia; which means that a toxin has accumulated in the blood above the toleration point"
~ **J. H. Tilden, M. D.**, from his book *Toxemia Explained*

"You can trace every sickness, every disease, and every ailment to a mineral deficiency"
~ **Linus Pauling, Ph. D.** (twice Nobel Laureate)

I believe main stream medicine is brilliant at treating symptoms and dealing with accidents and emergencies. Yet I also believe that by further scientific study in tracing symptoms of a chronic illness back to the source, could further medicine, reduce allot of suffering and reduce the NHS bill significantly.

The 3 possible causes of health issues we are going to look at are:

1. Toxemia, an accumulation of toxins from many different sources:

   - dental issues from mercury fillings and bacteria-riddled root canal fillings;
   - vaccine damage;
   - the side-effects of a cocktail of drugs and an excess of electromagnetic stress;
   - daily use of cosmetics containing too many toxic ingredients;
   - food or drinks containing harmful ingredients;
   - an emotional issue producing stress hormones over an extended period of time;
   - or a negative bacteria imbalance that excretes excess toxicity into your body.

2. Deficiency in Minerals/Vitamins or essential oils.

3. Structural alignment from back issues.

It doesn't sound too complicated, does it? The great news is all of these can be cleared or reduced by a considerable amount. The insight here is to look at each of these areas as feeding a possible health issue. One thing on its own may only compromise your immune system by maybe 5% but another issue adds another 5%. You can see how the feeds can soon add up, but also how it's possible to reduce the feeds.

Often the disease is the solution; it's your body's way of dealing with a toxic overload: the disease is not the problem, it is pointing toward the source. If you take in more toxins that your cells can excrete, you are going to have health issues, it is like if you don't take the trash out from your kitchen: your kitchen is going to stink.

If you get poisoned the body will have a fever, you may have a cold, you may have low energy and you may have joint issues and so on. You may be struggling to deal with your emotions and five minutes of depression or anger will compromise your immune system for six hours. You can try to live in ignorant bliss; in reality you will more than likely be living in ignorant pain. Good health is not about being disease free, it is about vibrant energy, because the body can compensate and deal with a whole load of toxins and problems. As you can start to see, this is not rocket science.

Let's go into more depth on these possible three main causes and how to clear or reduce these sources of many health issues.

1. TOXEMIA

Dental Issues

The Dangers of Mercury Poisoning
Silver fillings are around 50% mercury, an extremely potent neurotoxin. Mercury is one of the most poisonous substances on our planet. There is no safe level because even one atom of it in your body will do some damage. There is no debate about the toxicity of mercury and every knowledgeable scientist and health professional understands how poisonous it is. Dental mercury fillings were first exposed as

a health-compromising product in 1840, yet even today the Dental Association continues to say that the mercury released from these fillings is a safe amount.

The fact is, mercury in the body can make every health issue worse. Your dentist may disagree and say the amount of mercury released from an amalgam filling is so small as to have no negative effect—and I would probably agree that a few months of having an amalgam filling may not cause any harm—but these fillings are often in someone's mouth for years or even decades. This results in an accumulation of mercury in the body, so every time you chew your food or brush your teeth this stimulates more mercury to be released.

If you have a silver filling, mercury vapour is continually being released from it and that vapour enters the body and accumulates. Over time, the body loses its effectiveness in removing mercury and the accumulation accelerates.

The number and severity of symptoms depend on how many fillings you have, how long you've had them, and how often they are stimulated by eating, drinking and brushing your teeth.

The immune system works by destroying any 'non-self' invaders, meaning it has a code to destroy any cells it feels don't belong in your body. So when a mercury atom locks onto a healthy cell your immune system immediately identifies that cell as 'non self' and aims to kill and remove the contaminated cell. If that mercury is bonded to a nerve cell the result can be neurological disease, such as multiple sclerosis or seizures. Or if that mercury binds to a hormone, it can disrupt your endocrine function. Mercury can bind with almost any cell in your body and the result often creates an autoimmune disease.

In addition, because mercury is classified as a neurotoxin, it can also cause or contribute to emotional and psychological issues, such as depression, anxiety and mood swings.

If you need a filling I suggest choosing a white composite resin, which does not leak mercury, instead. If you are concerned because you already have a mercury filling there are now many mercury-free dentists around the world who can safely remove a mercury filling and replace it with a white composite. If you do find a dentist to do this please make sure they completely rubber-seal the tooth so all the mercury is completely removed and none of it is leaked into your body.

Afterwards it is useful to use a charcoal and NAC supplement, to help mop up any mercury that may be in the bloodstream. If there is a stubborn amount of mercury poisoning, I would recommend a chelation infusion, given by a qualified nurse, and a course of infrared saunas.

(For more information on this, you can read the biography of Dr. Tom McGuire, D.D.S., president of the Dental Wellness Institute and a leading authority on mercury detoxification, mercury amalgam fillings, chronic mercury poisoning and holistic dental wellness.)

The Hazards of Root Canal Fillings

The toxicity of root canals was jointly disclosed by the Mayo Clinic and Dr. Weston Price back in 1910. Price's textbook on root canals, published in 1922, upset the dental associations at that time and still does today.

The evidence clearly shows that toxins from anaerobic bacteria have the same ability as mercury to produce non-self cells, thus creating more autoimmune diseases. Price was concerned about the pathological bacteria found in root canal teeth.

Nearly all root canals contain colonies of bacteria that can cause major illnesses in your body. Even antibiotics won't help in these cases, because the bacteria are protected inside your dead tooth. When these bacteria migrate, via your bloodstream, to other areas of your body they can contribute to or cause more serious ailments such as heart and circulatory diseases, arthritis and rheumatism, and brain and nervous system diseases.

Again, like mercury fillings, there are solutions. You can have a replacement tooth made out of either white composite or porcelain or with a zirconium crown. This may cost more than a root canal filling but this research suggests it won't cost your health so much in the long term.

Did You Know your Teeth Have Nerve Connections with your Organs?

Have you ever been to the dentist and they hit a nerve, and you felt that pain throughout your whole body? Did you know your mouth has a reflexology chart, just like there is a foot reflexology chart? Each tooth has a connection to an organ through these nerves.

This is the reflexology chart for your teeth. What surprised me from working in health clinics around the world is that when we compared panoramic x-rays of the mouth an infected tooth almost always corresponded with the client's current health condition.

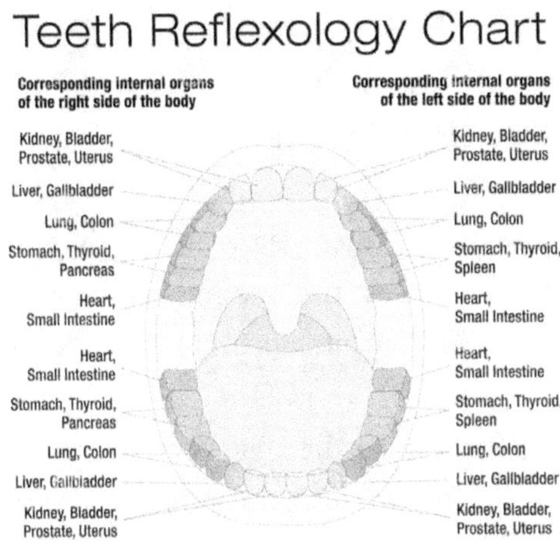

To use this to your advantage, find a local professional holistic dentist who does not believe in mercury fillings or root canal fillings. He or she will more than likely ask for you to have a panoramic x ray of your mouth which will help show up anything that needs to be seen in your teeth and your jaw. Then they will need to replace any amalgam fillings or root canal fillings with a safer option.

Your daily job is to look after your mouth, clean your teeth well and use a good mouthwash. Try coconut oil pulling; however make sure you only do it for about three minutes and then spit it out. The process pulls toxins from the mouth which, if left in your mouth too long, your body could reabsorb.

Vaccine Damage

This is a very challenging issue to write about because both sides say the complete opposite. I'm like many concerned people, looking for the truth. Robert De Niro as well as many well-known doctors have been campaigning and looking into the claims of hundreds of parents around the world who say their children's mental wellbeing literally changed overnight after having a vaccine.

More than ten million vaccines per year are given to children less than eighteen months old. At this age infants are at the greatest risk of certain adverse medical events, including high fevers and seizures.

Here is something to consider: In 1940 there were only two vaccinations, DTP and Smallpox. By 1980, this number rose to nine. Then by 2012 there are around 25 mandated vaccines often given 6 vaccine in one dose to children.

What most people fail to remember is that 1858 was the year of the Great Stink of London. Without a proper sewage system in London, sanitary levels were at an all-time low, in fact in the summer of that year London smelt so bad that the elite moved out of London en masse.

At this point the British government decided something had to be done and set about improving the sewage system in London. As it improved, many health issues also dramatically lessened. Then, years later, in the 1940s, when the worst of the sewage problems had been cleared up, many vaccines were introduced and claimed to have helped reduce so many illnesses. But, by simply cleaning up the sanitation, Britain saw a huge decrease in many illnesses before vaccines even came in.

You may be asking, what are the ingredients in these vaccines that so many doctors around the world are concerned about? Well, vaccines contain aluminium, formaldehyde, MSG, mercury and foetal cells. Many people are concerned that there has been no scientific trial comparing children who have had vaccines with children who haven't. To my mind this is a basic test of whether or not a drug is any good.

(If you would like to find out more, check out a film out called Vaxxed. If you're having a vaccine, I suggest asking your doctor for the list of ingredients in the vaccine and for the safety and side effect sheet, then make your own educated decision.)

EMF Radiation: "It's a No-Brainer"

Many people do not realise that mobile phone masts, smart meters, cordless phones, and Wi-Fi hubs can all emit electromagnetic radiation in the low microwave range of around (450–2100 MHz) research shows that this is safe. Which I agree to at a certain distance and a certain amount, but this technology is moving at a very fast pace and I do not believe we truly know the long term effect of EMR, and I believe people should be aware of simply solutions to reduce EMR if they wish to.

I met a person who designed and manufactured mobile phones and he told me he would not consider putting a mobile phone that was switched on next to his head.

If you're one of these people who is still in denial about this, please stand next to a mobile phone mast and feel the effect on your body; sit close to your Wi-Fi hub for 30 minutes and feel the effect; or talk on your mobile phone for 30 minutes with the phone next to your ear, and feel how it affects your head.

One of my clients lives in a block of flats surrounded by eighteen different Wi-Fi hubs and there is a mobile phone mast directly opposite her window on the roof of another block of flats. When we took some EMF readings they were off the scale. Even without my instruments I could feel what was like a mild burning to my skin. Her complaint was that she felt permanently anxious and found it pretty much impossible to sleep there.

I suggested she paint her flat with an EMF Radar Paint that captures and neutralises a lot of the radiation by earthing it through the plug socket or a cable that goes into the ground. In short, this paint makes a room feel like you're out in nature. Then we changed her Wi-Fi to Ethernet cable. She replaced her cordless home phone with a standard corded phone, and I suggested when she talked on her mobile either to switch it onto speaker and hold it away from her head or to use headphones. We then took further EMF readings, which were considerably reduced, and she reported back that she could sleep well in her own apartment and felt a lot more at ease.

The reason we feel EMF is because we have electrical charges in our cells. We are affected by electrical frequencies, which can have an effect on everything from our mood and our imagination to our physical health.

The point here is that the body can maybe cope with a small amount of EMF radiation and you might not feel much. Yet we live in this modern society where invisible radiation is all around us, so you can't really avoid it but you can reduce it and be smart. If you have sleep issues you might want to paint your bedroom with EMF paint.

Toxic Toiletries

My simple rule is that if you can't eat it, don't put it on your skin. Your skin absorbs whatever is applied to it and your body also eliminates waste through the skin. When you use antiperspirant deodorant you block up your pores, whereas you could just as easily use a natural deodorant that mops up the odour without pushing the natural waste back into your body.

U.S. researchers report that one in eight of the 82,000 ingredients used in personal care products are industrial chemicals, including carcinogens, pesticides, reproductive toxins and hormone disruptors.

Some toxic ingredients to watch out for in your bathroom products are: makeup with wrinkle-inducing parabens, sodium laureth sulphate, fluoride toothpastes, sunscreens containing cancer-causing benzophenones, triclosan siloxanes, formaldehyde-releasing preservatives, talc, dibutyl phthalate, DEA, BHA and BHT... and there are many more. In short, small amounts may not do much harm but the long-term use of them is very questionable.

My suggestion is simple: pop down to your health food store today and buy shampoo, toothpaste and skin cream without these toxic chemicals in.

DEFICIENCIES OF VITAMINS, MINERALS AND OMEGA 3 OILS

Did you know the average body has around fifteen million chemical reactions every single second?

Roughly 96% of the mass of the human body consists of just four elements: oxygen, carbon, hydrogen and nitrogen, a lot of which is in the form of water. The remaining 4% is a sparse sampling of the periodic table of elements, with around eighty trace minerals and twenty-three different vitamins.

You can quickly work out if you're missing a whole load of minerals, vitamins or essential omega oils as this will cause strain on your body's ability to work efficiently.

> *"Our bodies need at least 60 minerals each day in order to maintain a disease and ailment free state"*
> ~ **Dr Gary Price Todd**, M.D.

Did you know that the World Health Organization, the UK Ministry of Agriculture and Unicef have all found that the soil quality on farms worldwide has degenerated between 1910 and 2006? The average degeneration is North America -85%, South America -76%, Asia -76%, Africa -74%, Europe -72% and Australia -55%. Their findings show that even an organic diet is often severely lacking in nutrients.

> *"Research has shown micronutrient deficiency to be scientifically linked to a higher risk of overweight/obesity and other dangerous and debilitating diseases"*

To become micronutrient-sufficient on the standard American diet, based on FDA guidelines that the average body needs twenty-seven micronutrients per day, you would need to eat 27,575 calories per day!

The shocking news is that because our food is so deficient in minerals it means you have to eat a huge amount to get the same goodies out of it compared to a hundred years ago, so many overweight people are simply starved of minerals. In general we are overfed and undernourished.

Our bodies cannot survive without minerals, vitamins and essential omega oils which help maintain your immune system, healthy bones, enzyme function and cellular health. We will go into this more in the chapter on health supplements.

ISSUES WITH STRUCTURAL ALIGNMENT

If you have stubborn back pain that has been there a while, not only can it dampen your mood but it can also have a knock-on effect with a related organ depending on where the pain is located in your back.

Think of it this way: your brain talks to your body through a large speakerphone and your body talks to your brain through a large speakerphone. If there is a misalignment in your vertebrae and the nerve is pinched, that interferes with that communication. It's like putting a kink in a hosepipe which causes pressure: this then puts the system under stress, so it doesn't function so well. You then end up with faulty communication between your brain and body and this can cause a whole number of health issues. So keeping your spine healthy is a key factor for your overall health.

If you do have long-term back pain you will more than likely need a number of different strategies to get a really good result. Most people know about strengthening and stretching muscles and doing back rehabilitation classes like Pilates or going to see an osteopath, a chiropractor or a Bowen therapist, these are all great, yet I think most people with chronic back pain need a couple more things.

I have found the two most useful exercises are Somatics and the postural exercises from Egoscue. I will show you some of these movements in the on line videos.

Then there are other factors which we will go into later in this book; as mineral balancing has a role to play some lectin foods can cause inflammation, some foods and supplements can reduce inflammation. If there are bone issues from osteoporosis then exercises from Osteo-Strong can help, and your mindset plays a big role as well. In this book my aim is to bring all these factors together to help get you the best results.

My suggestions for your action steps this week, if you wish:

1. If you have any mercury fillings or root canal fillings, make an appointment to see a professional holistic dentist. Take extra care looking after your teeth on a daily basis.

2. Make a trip to your local health food store and treat yourself to some chemical-free soaps and cosmetics.

3. Reduce the levels of EMF in your environment using the suggestions above.

4. Try out a weekly online Pilates or Feldenkrais class and, if you feel the need, visit a local network chiropractor or osteopath for a general back care top up.

Prevention is far better than treatment.

Liquid Health

ONE OF THE EASIEST WAYS to improve your health is to start drinking more healthy drinks, reducing your intake of sugar-filled drinks and replacing them with drinks that not only taste great but which also have an immediate benefit for your health. The aim of this chapter is to introduce you to five types of incredible drinks to try out and to add one or two to your daily routine if you like them.

When you can create your own Tonic Bar at home, it means that when you make a drink for yourself you will know that some drinks can boost your brain power, some can give you extra energy and others can help relax you. The aim is for you to choose drinks according to your needs.

So are you ready to drink yourself healthy? The five drinks we are going to look are:

1. Making Water
2. Different Teas
3. Raw Milk
4. Chi, Jing and Shen drinks
5. Juicing/Smoothies.

DRINK 1: MAKING WATER

The first drink we are going to start with is water.

If you consider that the average adult human body is between 57-70% water, you may agree that getting a good source of clean water is a logical first step!

British tap water can contain hundreds of different man-made chemicals. It may look crystal clear, but tests reveal everything from trace amounts of benzotriazole and tolytriazole (chemicals found in dishwasher tablets) to pharmaceutical drugs such as antibiotics, antidepressants and contraceptive pills (which leak the female hormone oestrogen), heavy contaminates such as aluminium (which has been described as 'the silent killer,' known to increase the risk of Alzheimer's disease), and lead, which reaches your tap water through the corrosion of plumbing materials such as old pipes and can cause learning disabilities!

The number of trace chemicals in our tap water are too many to list. If I'm thirsty and there is nothing else to drink, I will drink tap water. But I would rather avoid drinking it.

My favourite way to make simple drinking water is to use a water distiller, which produces 100% clean water. The downside of this water is that some nutritionists say this is empty water and does not contain any beneficial minerals. I would also agree.

So my next step is to soak the distilled water in a jug with shungite rocks, which are rocks from Russia that help produce fullerenes, which help produce antioxidant molecules in the water. These rocks are very cheap to buy and will last for about 12 months. Then I add one teaspoon of Himalayan salt solution, or wet Celtic sea salt solution (also called sole), to every two litres of water.

Sole is a solution that contains over 80 different minerals and is totally different to using refined white salt that only contains sodium chloride and hardly anything else, which I would not recommend. This way you get 100% clean water with beneficial minerals, plus added antioxidants.

Once you bottle your water you can flavour it with slices of cucumber, lemon, ginger, fresh peppermint leaves or any other natural flavour you like. Or you can simply enjoy plain, natural, clean mineral water at a fraction of the price of bottled water.

Unlike water filters, where you have to keep changing costly filters, a water distiller involves just one initial cost of around £160 and it will last for years. I've had mine now for over five years and it works the same as when it was new. So you save money and you get great water, plus the environmental cost of transporting water bottles and disposing of them is reduced.

If you already have a good water filter, you can still soak your filtered water in the shungite rocks and add sole if you wish.

A great way to start your day is to have a large glass of warm water and lemon when you wake up, which helps fully hydrate your body.

DRINK 2: DIFFERENT TEAS

You know the phrase "it's time for tea"? Well how about adding some different teas to your tea collection? I often wonder why people mainly just drink standard tea when there are so many other amazing teas out there. My recommendation is get a nice teapot with an infuser, or tea tongs, and next time you are in a health food store or online experiment with some different teas.

Ginkgo tea is well known to help your brain function; Pardearco tea is a refreshing cleansing tea; Slippery Elm soothes the intestine; Hawthorn or Camomile tea is great to help you unwind and relax; Nettle tea is a good tonic for your liver; Borage tea or St John's Wort can help lift your mood and Matcha tea can give you a good energy boost. Matcha tea contains ten times the antioxidants of a regular green tea, with L-Theanine to boost brain power and ECGC to promote glowing skin.

You can sweeten green tea with a tiny amount of unrefined stevia powder, which some people really like.

DRINK 3: RAW MILK

Many health-conscious people seek out raw organic milk, as it's been drunk for thousands of years; nevertheless the government tell us it is dangerous to drink. What is the truth?

Public health officials warn us that raw milk poses the risk of transmitting bacteria such as E. coli and salmonella. While it is certainly possible to become sick from drinking contaminated raw milk, it is also possible to become sick from almost any contaminated food source.

I agree that drinking raw milk from cows kept indoors, fed on grains and pumped full of growth hormones and antibiotics, is not good for anyone. However, raw milk from organic cows that feed outdoors on grass is full of beneficial bacteria such as lactobacillus acidophilus and contains over 60 functional enzymes that improve your digestion. Raw milk can also improve the bioavailability of vitamins and minerals.

Also, if you are lactose intolerant when drinking pasteurized milk, you may find that if you start drinking a small amount of raw milk and build up slowly your milk intolerance may disappear. This is because lactase enzymes form when you digest raw milk. If you still have an issue with milk you can turn the raw milk into Kefir. This will give you the extra benefits of the friendly bacteria and some of my clients report this clears their milk intolerance, too. But milk simply does not suit many people, so really you need to consider what suits your body.

For myself, the biggest test after hearing both sides was trying some organic grass-fed raw milk and I was really surprised how good I felt from drinking it. Many supermarkets in the UK now stock unpasteurised cheese and butter and there are farms in the UK that do deliver raw milk. You'll need to research this in your local area or online.

DRINK 4: CHI, JING & SHEN DRINKS

Chinese medicine is based on three essential elements known as the Three Treasures. These are the essential energies sustaining human life: Chi, Jing and Shen.

Chi is easily obtained, it is the daily energy you derive from your food and drink and the air you breathe.

Jing is your deep source energy, it is the package of energy you were given at birth, like a battery in your inner core. You can see that some children have strong, robust energy so their Jing is strong, whereas some children are lacking in that strength so their Jing is weak.

Shen is your spiritual and emotional wellbeing, your connection to your higher self. When you see someone naturally happy most of the time their Shen is strong, whereas if a person is really down most of the time their Shen is low.

During our life, through overwork, stress, old age, excessive lust and illness, you can lose some of your potent Chi, Jing and Shen energy. However, there are a few powerful herbs that can replenish these energies, bringing you increased physical energy, overall body strength, calmness and balance and a better ability to cope with the everyday challenges of life. You can go to your local Chinese herbalist and get a formula perfectly made up for you, or you can test out some of these herbs and feel for yourself what they do. I find it very beneficial knowing the effect of each herb for myself.

Some Chi herbs you could try are Ginseng, Astragulus, and Maca. Some Jing herbs you could try include He Shou Wu, Eucommia, Morinda, and Deer Antler. Shen herbs you could try include Cordceps or Reishi.

All these words may sound weird to you. If they do, don't worry; keep your mind open and see it as a learning experience. I first tried a Jing herb drink when I was rebuilding my strength after healing from cancer. My energy was at an all-time low: as soon as I had one of these drinks it was like drinking an everlasting smile! My friend Aradhana and I came up with a drink called Immortal Cheer which was full of these Jing herbs.

Most of these herbs are quite bitter to taste, so there is a bit of skill needed to make them taste amazing. The trick is to blend something bitter with, for example, some cashew nuts to make it creamy, and then add some Goji Berries for some fruitiness and sweetness.

In our online course I will show you how to make an Immortal Cheer and many other similar drinks using Chi, Jing and Shen Herbs. I will share with you the best time of day to drink these tonic herbs and also the best places to buy your herbs from, because the quality varies so much.

The nice thing with tonic herb drinks is that when you're feeling a bit run down and you've been burning the candle at both ends these drinks can really replenish you. It's not like a coffee rush or high, they provide deep replenishing energy.

Once you have this knowledge you can judge for yourself if you need one a day to top up your energy or just when you feel the need. This is like medicine for the soul.

DRINK 5: GREEN SMOOTHIES AND JUICING

Your mother used to say eat your greens and eat your vegetables and no nutritionist disagrees with that. Yet if the thought of eating a huge pile of vegetables seems hard work, juicing is the easy way to get your five-a-day in one drink and often people are really surprised by how tasty these drinks are. There are many different ways of juicing different fruits and vegetables. Jason Vale's book, "Super Juice Me" suggests some of the best combinations.

The difference between juicing and a smoothie is that juicing extracts the juice from the fruits and vegetables whereas smoothies blend the whole food, so you get all the fibre as well as the juice. Both are great, they are just slight variations. The key point here is to inspire you to have a good juicer and blender at home so you can make your own fresh fruit and vegetable juices and smoothies.

Also you may have heard of all these superfood green powder blends that contain ingredients like wheat grass, barley grass, spirulina and chlorella. They're like a power pack of nutrients and I like adding some of these ingredients to my smoothies or juices.

My favourite juice, both for flavour and for how it makes me feel, is carrot, kale, ginger, Co Yo Coconut Yoghurt and some super green powder blend.

My favourite smoothie is a blend of coconut milk, mango, banana, Co Yo Coconut Yoghurt, ginger, cayenne pepper and some super green powder.

If you're in general good health, most combinations are great. However if you're healing a health condition you may need to limit the amount of sweet fruit to the absolute minimum as bad bacteria and cancer can feed on fruit sugars. So the skill is knowing when you need discipline to stick to a low level of sweet fruit. In the online training I will give you lots of drink recipes.

My suggestions for this week,
if you wish:

1. Look at how you can improve the quality of water you already drink using the recommendations above.

2. There are different views on raw milk; some people agree it's good for you but in many countries it is illegal. If you're interested please look into this for yourself and come to your own conclusions.

3. See if you can try three different herbal teas this week.

4. Try one Chi tonic drink, one Jing tonic drink and one Shen tonic drink and see if you can notice the effect on your body.

5. Try adding one juice or smoothie per day and add a super green powder blend to the mix.

The drinks you have on a daily basis can be the simplest form of medicine or the slowest form of poison. My final tip is don't be scared to try out some new ingredients. It's only by trying new ingredients that you can truly find out what works for you.

Food For Life

> " Don't dig your grave with
> your own knife and fork."
> ~ OLD ENGLISH PROVERB

IMAGINE IF YOU WERE ABLE to condense time, from the beginning of the Homo Sapiens species to the present day, into a 24-hour period. It is only in the last seven minutes that we have drastically changed the way we live and eat!

In this sudden change we have forgotten a lot of the simple basics of healthy eating. In this chapter we are going to combine a basic understanding of what our ancestors ate for thousands of years with the best of the food and recipes we have today.

Eating habits around the world are based on anything from deeply-held beliefs to following the latest fashion diet. Food can be one of the main causes of so many health conditions, from diabetes and cancer to heart disease, obesity and many others. So it makes logical sense that food can also be part of the solution to many, many health issues.

Yet, like many other people, you may be confused and overwhelmed with all the conflicting information. Maybe you saw someone succeed on a particular diet and tried it for yourself but it had no effect. I believe this is because everyone is slightly different: for example we have different jobs and live in different climates; there are four different human blood types and we each have different metabolisms. These factors and others mean we each have slightly different nutritional needs. That's why one way or one diet does not fit all.

So over the years I've developed nine Healthy Food Factor guidelines to help our clients select healthy options when they are eating out or cooking at home that give their body the nourishment it needs with enjoyment and satisfaction.

If you are a vegetarian or meat eater you can personalise these Food Factor Guidelines to eat more healthily.

The result of following these guidelines is more vibrant energy during the day, your emotions will feel more in balance, you'll sleep more easily and you'll naturally return to your perfect weight. This will also help reduce symptoms of most health issues. So the nine Food Factor Guidelines to eating your way back to health are:

1. Keep it Simple
2. Food Energetics
3. Is Meat Good or Bad For You?
4. Intolerance and Mineral Testing

5. Fat Facts

6. Grain Gains

7. Intelligent Eating

8. Balancing your Gut Bacteria

9. Mindful Eating

The insight to consider for this chapter is that when someone is diagnosed with a health issue, that health issue did not happen overnight. It's more than likely it took years to develop. Long-term bad eating habits can creep up on people and their first sign of a health issue may be a major disease. If you do have a health issue, it can take a lot of skill and time to restore your health: it's almost like your body has been looking after you on autopilot and now it's asking you to work with it in partnership. Yet most of your cells regenerate within 90 days, so if you apply the health tips in this book, you could literally be a new person in just 90 days!

Imagine it this way: you are looking at goldfish in a goldfish bowl. If the water is clean and fresh the goldfish will be healthy; if that water gets sludgy, murky and filled with crap, the goldfish will become unwell. The water of the fish bowl is like your blood: if you fill it with unhealthy fats, processed foods, chemically-enhanced foods and so on, it will make your blood stickier and less effective in all the jobs it naturally does on a daily basis.

Once you understand these nine guidelines you will be able to make healthy, delicious choices. You will be able to look at any recipe book or a menu in a restaurant and know what's the best for you and why. You will have the best of both worlds: food that is tasty and that you love and that is also healthy.

1. KEEP IT SIMPLE

There are many different diets around the world: Blood Group diets, Caveman diets, the New Atkins diet, Food Combining, Vegan, Metabolic Typing, Raw Food diets, Alkalising diets, and many more. You may be asking why people around the world are getting beneficial results with what seem on the surface to be totally different diets.

One answer is the common factor between most of the diets where people get great results: they all leave out or reduce refined grains, refined oils, pasteurised dairy, refined sugars, artificial sweeteners and processed foods laden with chemicals.

When food has added chemicals, it can make you want more, even when you're full. They will make you enjoy eating poor-quality foods. Plus, these taste-enhancing chemicals cause people to become habitually addicted to the food they eat, which sadly transcends their logic and intelligence.

The secret is making improvements bit by bit. If you eat pasteurised dairy products, look for some unpasteurised dairy products where the digestive enzymes have not been destroyed. Instead of using white processed sugar use coconut sugar, which is a more complex sugar that keeps your blood sugar level more balanced. Instead of chemically-enhanced processed packet meals, choose fresh organic packet meals. If you're in a supermarket buying aspartame or sugar-filled fruit yogurt, you could choose a natural sugar-free yogurt and add a sugar-free jam. Even better, you could get a coconut yogurt which is dairy-free.

It's about being smart and looking at labels when you're shopping. If it looks like a NASA scientist designed this ready meal, think twice about it and choose the natural option. The great thing is today most supermarkets and cafés have healthy options. I love Prêt A Manger organic coffee and natural food cafés where I can enjoy fresh carrot and ginger juice, fresh soups, fresh quinoa salads and so much more. The point is that as you develop the eight other Food Factor Guidelines they will all come together to help you make healthy choices personal to you.

2. FOOD ENERGETICS

I learnt this when I was about 20. At that time, my job was mainly loading or unloading lorries and food simply meant I could do my grafting. When my nutrition teacher told me to listen to the effect of a meal on my body after eating, I thought she was nuts. I thought food equals energy and that was it. Little did I know!

> *"Listen to your body's whispers; otherwise you will be forced to listen to your body's screams."*

When you have a meal or any snack, you need to ask yourself questions like this:

How do you feel one hour later, two hours later? How has that food affected your energy levels? Has it been heavy or light on your digestion? Has it given you energy and strength or has it made you sleepy? Has it made you feel cold or warm? Does your head feel foggy or do you feel clear and alert? Has it had a contracting, grounding effect or left you feeling like you can't sit still?

Instead of giving you a long list of the effects of this food and that, it is simpler to start paying more attention to how you feel after you have eaten some food. The more you listen to your body's whispers, the more intelligent choices you'll make and the healthier you'll feel.

Plus you can use this universal skill on any nutritional advice. As you will probably be trying some new foods and recipes, this skill is your barometer of whether they're right for you or not.

3. IS MEAT GOOD OR BAD FOR YOU?

If you are a meat eater, how much meat is good for you? Meat contains a power pack of nutrition, yet excessive meat consumption is now related to some cancers.

The most logical explanation I can give you is to compare a human gastrointestinal (GI) tract (the tract that starts in the mouth and finishes at the anus) with that of a typical herbivore (plant eater) and a typical carnivore (meat eater).

We will use the cow and tiger as examples but all plant eaters and all meat eaters share similar characteristics. For accuracy, scientists measure the length of the GI tract then measure the length of the animal's torso and divide them to give a ratio. The tiger's ratio = 3:1, the cow's ratio = 12:1 and a human ratio = 10:1.

The tiger's ratio shows that its GI tract is short. This enables it to digest meat quickly. All the essential nutrients will be absorbed but the meat does not have time to putrefy. This is an important fact to acknowledge: meat will putrefy at 37°C, which is normal body temperature, so meat eaters have a shorter GI tract to avoid the growth of bad bacteria.

The cow's ratio shows it has a much longer GI tract: this is because grass does not putrefy, so it can take as long as it wants to absorb all the nutrients. The human ratio of 10:1 is closer to the cow's ratio of 12:1, but nowhere near the tiger's ratio of 3:1. This shows that our digestive system is made to eat mainly plant food, with a small amount of meat if you wish.

Currently, in the western world, many people eat meat every day. Some people even eat it at every meal. Our bodies are simply not designed to such large quantities of meat.

Our teeth are another good indicator of how much meat we should eat. These are our tools for eating. They show clearly what we are designed to eat. Tigers, along with other meat eaters, have pointy teeth that are far apart. Cows and other plant eaters have teeth that are flat on top and close together. Humans have four canine teeth which are slightly pointy but the rest are flat and they are all close together. So again we are far more similar to the herbivores than the carnivores but still in-between.

On top of this, processed meats such as bacon or salami contain sodium nitrates which kill off spores of Clostridium Botulinum. Yet the sodium nitrates are also harmful to you and increase your risk of bowel cancer. Did you know eating two rashers of bacon has the equivalent effect on your health of smoking four cigarettes? Also if you barbecue your meat and it turns black this produces a chemical called PA8H, which is a known carcinogen.

If your choice is to eat meat, the Food Factor Guideline is to choose organic, unprocessed meat which, if eaten in moderation and cooked without burning, is a power pack of nutrients for you. Meat is sometimes given a bad name yet it can also be a medicine eaten as an organic bone broth—a powerhouse super food known to help improve everything from digestion and immunity to joint flexibility. Some people really do well on more meat than others. For example, 'O' blood types and those with 'protein' types in metabolic typing thrive with meat in their diet. Again it is about listening to your body, not what is written in a fashion magazine.

4. INTOLERANCE AND MINERAL TESTING

Often a magazine or newspaper will say one particular food is a healthy choice, yet it does not mean it is healthy for everyone. The insight here is that one person's food can be another person's poison.

My suggestion for this Food Factor Guideline is for you to get a comprehensive intolerance test. There is a huge difference between allergies and intolerances: allergies can have big reaction, e.g. a rash or swelling can occur, whereas intolerances are more subtle and may hardly be noticed. You may only experience a small negative effect, such as bloating, tiredness, foggy thinking, digestive issues or mild symptoms of IBS.

On our website we show you how and where to get your intolerance tests. Once you have the test results, you can replace the foods that cause you these slight intolerances and increase the foods that nourish your body.

One issue with these intolerance tests is that they are a soft science. Intolerances can be very subtle: they can change and can often be corrected by leaving out the offending foods for a period of time, by addressing the vitamin and mineral imbalance, or by having a detox. For these reasons it is hard to get 100% accuracy, yet the tests do provide clear indications of intolerances.

Sometimes a test simply shows the client that a specific food shouldn't dominate their diet but a small amount may be fine. This is where your Food Energetics practice comes in so you can feel the effects yourself once the test has given you a good indication of what to look out for.

The other important test I recommend is a mineral test. When we re-test the same sample we get back pretty much 100% the same results, meaning the mineral test shows a lot more clearly which minerals are out of balance in your body. Correcting your mineral imbalances is one of the key factors to your overall health.

For example, often a sign of potassium deficiency is pain down the right side of the body. Signs of a magnesium deficiency are finding it hard to deal with stress and not being able to relax. You may also suffer from cramps in the leg, or constipation.

Iodine often comes up as a deficiency and this can cause dry skin issues, brain fog and memory issues. Common chemical compounds such as bromine (used as a fire retardant and often added to baking ingredients and used in plastics) displace iodine from the body. One mineral, vitamin or chemical compound often has a knock-on effect on another.

Then there are also 70 fulvic minerals that may not show up in your cells yet they show up in your gut bacteria and for some people this is a piece of the puzzle they were looking for. You can get your fulvic minerals from food supplements such as Shilajit.

Once the test has shown which minerals you need, you can look for certain foods that are high in that mineral. For example, if your sodium is high and your potassium is low drinking carrot juice, which is rich in potassium, will help rebalance this. By taking a chromium and vanadium supplement you can reduce sugar cravings, and these minerals often help diabetics.

Mineral deficiency can also cause weight gain as some people have this band of excess weight around their belly and they find it impossible to shift, no matter what diet or exercise they do. This could be caused by too many heavy metals in their body from sources such as aluminium saucepans, polluted air, kitchen foil, spray-on deodorants etc. Then once these heavy metals are in your bloodstream, your body will protect you from them by wrapping them in a layer of fat. Certain minerals can help clear these heavy metals from your body but if you're deficient in them your body cannot do the cleaning up. Sometimes adding in the correct mineral can help you get back to your natural bodyweight.

The mineral balances in your body have a huge part to play in everything from your physical to your emotional health. If you would like to research this more, Lawrence Wilson M.D., who has written a book called "Nutritional Balancing with Hair Analysis", is one of the leading experts in this field. We will cover more in our on line training.

5. FAT FACTS

By the 1960s, the American Heart Association was recommending that people reduce their fat intake. The average American learned that carbs were good while fat was bad, which more than likely set off a sugar addiction, leading to an obesity epidemic. This shows decades of government health advice, particularly with regard to heart disease, cholesterol levels and the consumption of fats and oils, has been plain wrong.

Our bodies need fat. More specifically, they need healthy fats. While bad fats can increase your risk of certain diseases, good fats protect your brain and heart. In fact, healthy fats—such as omega-3s—are vital to your physical and emotional health. Understanding how to include more healthy fat in your diet can help improve your mood, boost your brain and memory function, increase your emotional wellbeing and even trim your waistline.

Often Grannies know best. In this case, those Grannies who cooked with goose fat, butter, ghee or coconut oil (depending on from what part of the world they came) instinctively knew what was right.

The key point to realise is that coconut oil or similar saturated fats are great for heavy frying; rapeseed oils are good for light frying and olive, pumpkin and avocado oils are ideal for dressings and dips.

This is because when you heat oils such as vegetable oils, olive oil or sunflower oil at high temperatures the nourishing parts of the oil break down and turn into chemicals called aldehydes, which have been linked to illnesses including cancer, heart disease and dementia.

Very few oils are stable at high temperature. Only oils such as coconut oil and ghee are stable at high cooking temperatures. The fats to reduce or avoid are from fried foods cooked in hydrogenated oils.

Many other oils are also beneficial for your body. Avocados, for example, are rich in monounsaturated fats, raise levels of good cholesterol and are also packed with the benefits of vitamin E, which helps prevent free radical damage, boosts immunity and acts as an anti-aging nutrient for your skin. Coconut oil is an effective anti-inflammatory, anti-fungal food and can help reduce symptoms of arthritis.

Tips when buying olive oil: check the harvesting date on the label; if it's labelled as "light," or a "blend," it isn't virgin quality; and finally, look for dark bottles as they protect the oil from oxidation.

When buying butter, aim to buy unpasteurised, grass-fed butter which contains more omega-3 oils and vitamins, more MCT, more CLA and many more beneficial nutrients compared to butter from cows fed on animal feed. Millions of years of evolution have tended to get things right: margarine has now proved not to be better for you than butter. In fact, many studies have proven that margarine is a cocktail of harmful fats that is best avoided.

In a nutshell, enjoy your good fats, reduce your bad fats, and cook with the right oils at the right temperatures.

6. GRAIN GAINS

Humans have been consuming grains for the last 10,000 years. It is only since the 1960s, with the introduction of draft wheat, the practice of regularly spraying wheat with Roundup and the way grains are refined and treated today, that health issues have been on the rise. I consider that two of the most common foods that contribute to many health issues are white refined flour and white refined sugar: if you can reduce or avoid these two foods you'll notice the benefits quickly.

1% of Americans now have celiac disease, and 6-8% have non-celiac sensitivity. When people with celiac disease eat wheat, the immune system in the gut mistakenly assumes that the gluten proteins are foreign invaders and mount an attack. However the immune system doesn't only attack the Lectin gluten proteins, it also attacks the gut lining itself, leading to degeneration of the intestinal lining, leaky gut, and inflammation.

Yet if whole grains are sprouted and fermented, the negative effects of the lectins are reduced. Think of it this way: a grain seed needs to lock in all of its nutrition, maybe until the coming year, to protect their seeds, so when you soak or sprout grains the more nutrients you release and the easier they are to digest. Studies suggest they produce less, if any, sensitivity in people who have a mild sensitivity to gluten.

Grain tips:

- When you're shopping, look for organic sprouted flour. Most health food stores do now stock this.

- If you are on a restrictive diet and are avoiding all grains, you can use vegetables in place of grains in many dishes. Try cabbage or sea spaghetti instead of pasta, or sliced sweet potatoes or kombu strips instead of lasagne sheets.

- You can also make breads with grain-free flours like coconut flour, gram flour or almond flour, or make linseed crackers if you're looking for that crunchy crisp texture.

7. INTELLIGENT EATING

A hummingbird will sip the nectar from many different flowers: I applied this insight to all the different diets out there. I see intelligence in all of them and if you are able to take the best information from any diet and then apply the other guidelines in this chapter you will be able to extract the best information and then personalize it for you.

From a raw food diet, you have enzyme-rich foods and foods containing a high concentration of nutrients. When you eat raw chocolate, compared to eating standard chocolate, not only does it taste better, you can feel the endorphin effect so much more. When you eat fresh kale crisps they knock the socks off standard crisps, being so much tastier and many times better for you. For some people too much raw food does not suit them but for others it is the perfect diet, so discover for yourself which are your favourite raw food recipes. I highly recommend buying a dehydrator to make things like kale crisps and linseed crackers. A great recipe book to start with is "Eat Smart Eat Raw" by Kate Magic.

The wisdom in vegetarian cooking is to eat plenty of vegetables: our bodies are designed to eat a higher proportion of plant-based foods. Once you have discovered cookbooks like "Gaia Kitchen: Vegetarian Recipes for Family and Community" you will love vegetarian food because it simply tastes so good. Because it feels light and healthy on your body you'll naturally crave more of these tasty recipes.

The wisdom from metabolic typing is that different ratios of fats, carbohydrates and protein suit different body types. This is a really clever system and you can easily do an online test to discover your metabolic type. You can establish the ratio of fats, protein and carbs per plateful that should suit your body and then use your food energetics to double-check if it's right for you.

The golden nectar from the hummingbird diet is to take any diet and use the principles of food energetics to test it out and personalize it to your body's needs.

8. BALANCING YOUR GUT BACTERIA

The average 20-year-old today will have already had eighteen different courses of antibiotics and much of our food is contaminated with low levels of antibiotics used in farming. Perhaps not surprisingly this can have a negative effect on our gut bacteria. Achieving the right gut bacteria balance can strengthen your immune system and uplift your mood and energy levels. Getting it wrong will weaken your immune system and can lead to weight issues, mood swings and often feeling tired.

One of the best ways to increase your friendly gut bacteria is to make your own fresh fermented vegetables, or fresh kefir that will outperform most of the expensive probiotics you can buy in a health food shop. These fermented foods prime your gut bacteria, promoting the second meal effect, slowing your digestion and helping you absorb much more goodness from your food.

9. MINDFUL EATING

If you eat slowly and in a more relaxed fashion, your digestive system is going to work a lot better. The French understand this and take their time enjoying their meals: eating is a leisurely enjoyable experience in France. French life expectancy is ninth in the world and I believe this leisurely approach to eating contributes a great deal. If you're eating when you're stressed, your digestive system can't work properly. It is that simple: if you relax while you eat it is better for your physical and emotional health, and avoid over eating as this stresses the body out.

The secret to slowing down your eating is to use all your senses. Savour the smells coming off your food; observe how it looks; notice the texture and flavour of what enters your mouth.

As you can see, all of these Food Factor Guidelines will help you to eat yourself healthy and, instead of being rigid guidelines or a strict diet, you can personalise them to you.

My suggestions for you this coming week:

1. Make an extra effort to keep it simple: reduce or avoid refined, processed foods and look to increase unrefined foods. Have a clear out in your kitchen and stock up with healthy essentials (we will go more deeply into this in our online course).

2. Try to become more aware of the Food Energetics: that is, the effect the food has on you after you have eaten it.

3. If you do eat meat, aim this week to buy organic and eat the right ratio of meat for your body.

4. You can purchase an intolerance test and a mineral test from our website to help take the guesswork out of what foods to reduce or increase in your diet and what selective minerals your body needs.

5. Increase your good fats, decrease the bad fats and cook with fats that are stable at high temperatures as suggested.

6. If it suits your body, try to add some sprouted flour products and experiment to see if you notice a difference in using them. Take any existing health conditions into consideration, as sometimes it is best to leave out grains for a period of time until symptoms are cleared.

7. Practice looking at any recipe book to see if you can now extract the best information from any recipe or know what to ask for in a restaurant to personalise the options to you.

8. Work to strengthen your gut bacteria with freshly-made fermented foods or buy a kefir starter kit.

9. Take your time when you eat and enjoy your food through all your senses by seeing, smelling and tasting your food.

In our online training course we will give you a PDF handout of how to create an incredible, tasty weekly menu plan. We will give you a shopping list and lots of recipes aligned with helping reduce symptoms of an autoimmune disease and what may help diet-wise if you're recovering from cancer. Or, if you're simply interested in prevention, this information can make that difference, too.

Also if you would like some inspiring cookbooks, these are some of my favourites: Jason Vale "Super Fast Food", Yotam Ottolenghi "Plenty", "Gaia's Kitchen" with Julia Ponsonby, "Deliciously Ella Every Day" by Ella Woodward, "Raw Living—Detox Your Life" and "Eat the High Energy Way" by Kate Magic, and Amelia Freer "Cook Nourish Glow".

The essence of this chapter is simply this: fall in love with healthy food that nourishes you on every level to feel consistently satisfied, energised and balanced, helping you live your life to the fullest. Before you know it, you'll be cooking a whole load of new recipes that you not only love but that also support your health and life in ways you can't imagine.

I invite you to discover the positive effects of eating healthy for yourself. Become motivated to discover those foods and recipes that you.

Power Supplements

"The six best doctors anywhere, and no one can deny, are sunshine, water, rest, air, exercise and diet."

~ WAYNE FIELDS

THE WAY WE EAT AND live today is so vastly different to seventy years ago. Our bodies are often under the strain of many new chemicals and toxins in our food. Excessive quantities of refined sugars cause excess amounts of insulin, leading to inflammation and weight gain. The food we eat is so vastly deficient in vitamins and minerals compared to what our grandparents were brought up on. Food intolerances such as intolerance to wheat can also rob you of valuable nutrients, setting off a chain reaction of unbalancing different nutrients, which in turn unbalances your mood and possibly leads to health issues.

For all these reasons, I believe it is a necessity to take some health supplements, although I prefer to keep this to a minimum.

These days too many people knock back so-called health supplements without really knowing if they need them and not really caring about the quality or effectiveness of the supplement they choose. Sometimes a supplement may cause a further imbalance, hindering the healing process because too much of one mineral, for example, can knock another mineral out of balance.

The five key health supplements we are going to focus on in this chapter are listed below. This combination of nutrients can be used for general health and wellbeing:

1. Trace Minerals
2. B Vitamins
3. Vitamin D3 and K2
4. Omega 3 Oils
5. Antioxidant Nrf2 Protandim

Most importantly, you need to get the correct supplements from the right source. Just as you wouldn't put bad fuel in your car, you don't want a poor quality supplement in your body. A lot of supplements are literally a waste of time and are full of fillers or lubricates such as magnesium stearate.

When we recommend a health supplement we suggest finding it in a liquid form or food state supplement if possible, as this is more likely to be absorbed and utilised better by your body.

Also, if your body needs a specific vitamin, mineral or oil, see if you can first find it in its natural form (e.g. for iodine take a kelp supplement or eat more seaweed, or get vitamin B5 from royal jelly, and so on).

1. TRACE MINERALS

"You can trace every sickness, every disease, and every ailment to a mineral deficiency"
~ **Linus Pauling,** Ph.D. (twice Nobel Laureate)

We'll start with trace minerals because this is one of the most important nutrient groups. Vitamins can be useless or sometimes even harmful without minerals, and the multitude of chemical reactions between vitamins and minerals are finely balanced.

For example, there is a sodium/potassium balance, a magnesium/calcium balance and iodine only works with its co-factor selenium. There are so many other pairings that rely on each other to work.

The problem is, our soil and food are severely deficient in minerals, a devastating change from as little as seventy years ago that causes many imbalances in people's internal chemistry. An interesting example is Jamaica, which has one of the lowest levels of Boron in their soil in the world due to excessive sugar farming and chemical fertilizers. Jamaica also has one of the highest levels of arthritis in the world. Bone analysis of arthritic joints and nearby bones show half the Boron content of healthy joints and synovial fluid—the connection is clear.

For general health we recommend a broad spectrum plant-based mineral supplement. For any chronic health issues we do suggest taking a mineral test to identify your specific needs.

2. B VITAMINS

B vitamins are an essential that many people are lacking in. B vitamins can help you ease stress, reduce anxiety, reduce depression, aid memory, relieve PMS, reduce the risk of heart disease and boost your metabolism.

People at risk of multiple B vitamin deficiencies include older adults, vegetarians or vegans, and those with alcoholism and heart failure. People also take a B-Complex supplement to increase energy, support brain health, enhance mood, improve memory, and ease stress.

All B vitamins help your body convert food (carbohydrates) into fuel (glucose), which the body uses to produce energy as well as for healthy skin, hair, and eyes, proper functioning of the nervous system and liver, a healthy digestive tract, making red blood cells which carry oxygen throughout the body, and making sex- and stress-related hormones in the adrenal glands.

The eight B vitamins are B1, B2, B3, B5, B6, B7, B9 and B12

B1, also known as Thiamine, helps regulate your appetite and support your metabolism.

B2, also known as Riboflavin, helps keep your skin, eyes and nervous system healthy.

B3, also known as Niacin, helps regulate the nervous and digestive systems. Niacin has a long history of helping treat symptoms of anxiety and depression very effectively. A strong property of niacin is its ability to relax the muscle tissue of arteries, which increases their diameter. This process, called vasodilatation, leads to increased blood flow and can help reduce blood pressure.

B5, also known as Pantothenic acid, helps with the proper functioning of the nervous system. B5 is widely known to be beneficial in treating serious mental disorders like chronic stress and anxiety.

B6 helps the body make several neurotransmitters, chemicals that carry signals from one nerve cell to another. It is needed for normal brain development and function, and helps the body make the hormones such as serotonin, which influence mood, and melatonin, which helps regulate the body clock.

B7, also known as Biotin. This helps with improving metabolism, tissue maintenance, healthy skin and weight issues, and offers relief from heart problems

B9, also known as Folic Acid or Brewer's Yeast, helps lower the risk of heart disease, stroke, and birth defects. This vitamin is especially important for women who are pregnant since it supports the growth of the baby and prevents neurological birth defects.

B12, also known as Cobalamin. Signs of vitamin B12 deficiency are dizziness, vertigo, forgetfulness, muscle weakness, pale skin, numbness and shaking in the hands. B12 can help address those issues.

As you can see, B vitamins play a huge role in your health and wellness. From the list above, notice if you suffer from any of the symptoms of B Deficiency. If you do you can see if a B-Complex supplement would reduce these symptoms, or you could increase your intake of foods rich in vitamin B, such as avocados, yoghurt, lentils, chlorella, greens, spinach, grains, nuts, royal jelly, fish, eggs and meats.

3. VITAMIN D3 AND K2

Vitamin D deficiency is a worldwide public health problem. We get vitamin D from sunshine, which allows our skin to create the vitamin in the form of vitamin D3. We all recognise the health warnings about staying out too long in the sun, yet these health warnings don't normally state that too little sunshine is also harmful. The problem is, we drive to work in our cars, park in an underground car park and then sit inside all day, getting little or no sunshine.

Current research has implicated vitamin D deficiency as a major factor in the pathology of at least seventeen varieties of cancer as well as heart disease, stroke, hypertension, autoimmune diseases, diabetes, depression, chronic pain, osteoarthritis, osteoporosis, muscle weakness, muscle wasting, birth defects, periodontal disease, and more.

> *"This is like the Holy Grail of cancer medicine; vitamin D produced a drop in cancer rates greater than that for quitting smoking, or indeed any other countermeasure in existence."*
> ~ **Dennis Mangan,** clinical laboratory scientist.

Adequate vitamin D levels can prevent bones from becoming thin, brittle, or malformed. It is linked with the prevention of osteoporosis.

It is best to get twenty minutes of sun on your full body every day to get your D3: otherwise you can have a vitamin D3 and K2 supplement or use a vitamin D lamp. K2 helps the absorption of D3, so if you do get a D3 supplement check if it has K2 in as well. This vitamin is vital to your immune system; make sure you get enough each day.

4. OMEGA 3 OIL

Omega 3 Oil has been increasingly shown to have beneficial effects on cardiovascular health, inflammation, mental health, and neurodegenerative diseases. Yet throughout our five million years of evolution, our diets have been abundant in seafood and other sources of omega 3 long chain fatty acids (EPA eicosapentaenoic & DHA docosahexaenoic) but relatively low in omega 6 seed oils.

Research suggests that our hunter-gatherer ancestors consumed omega 6 and omega 3 fats in a ratio of roughly 1:1. Today most people eat way too much food containing omega 6 fatty acids and way too little of omega 3 essential oils. Some estimates today say some people are consuming omega 6 to 3 ratio to around 16:1.

A high imbalance of Omega-6 intake can increase inflammation and has been associated with violence and depression, while Omega-3s can improve all sorts of mental disorders like depression, even schizophrenia and bipolar disorder.

Another problem with a high Omega-6 intake is the fact that the double bonds in the fatty acid molecules are very reactive to heat.

They tend to react with oxygen, forming chain reactions of free radicals that can cause damage to molecules in cells, which is one of the mechanisms behind aging.

The advice is to consider your Omega-6 intake by reducing or avoiding processed heated seed- and vegetable oils which are high in Omega-6. Sunflower, Corn, Soybean and Cottonseed oils are by far the worst as they have very little if any omega 3 and very high in omega 6. I recommend avoiding these especially in cooking.

Butter, ghee, coconut oil, lard, palm oil are all relatively low in Omega-6 and are much more stable in cooking.

If you're looking to strengthen your immune system, improve your mood, reduce inflammation, relief from painful periods and improve your joint health. One option would be to consider adding in a high quality cod liver oil supplement which is high in omega 3, but make sure it is of high quality and has not gone rancid.

Even more effective than a Fish Oil would be a Krill Oil combined with Astaxanthin supplement, as Krill oil is super rich in omega 3 and EPA and DHA and is highly absorbable and is less likely to go rancid.

Astaxanthin is the red-orange pigment that can be found in crustaceans and microalgae and has been proven to support the heart, brain, eyes, skin and immune system and provide pain relief. There have been over 400 peer-reviewed studies on AstaReal and Astaxanthin, AstaReal is the form of Astaxanthin with 50 human studies on its database including 23 double-blind placebo controlled trials that back its use. Research shows that Krill Oil and Astaxanthin work well together.

If your vegetarian or vegan hemp oil or flaxseed oil is the preferred plant based alternative to krill oil and has almost a perfect balance profile of omega 3, 6 and 9 fatty acids.

5. ANTIOXIDANT NRF2 PROTANDIM

The Washington State University stated that Nrf2 Protandim "Is potentially the most extraordinary therapeutic and preventative breakthrough in the history of medicine" And this is backed up with 23 peer-reviewed studies published on pub med so it is medically proven.

Nrf2 is a protein in your cell that communicates to the Nucleus of the cell, to say "Hey boss we've got allot of toxins to clear up, can we produce some of our own glutathione to help clean this up." Glutathione is your body's natural antioxidant and is extremely effective at clearing up free radicals. Over time most people's antioxidants drop and their free radicals increase.

What Dr. Joe Mc Cord worked out from decades of research in Nutrigenomics. Nutrigenomics is the scientific study of the interaction of nutrition on genes, especially with regard to the prevention or treatment of disease. He discovered that by combining Milk Thistle, Bacopa, Ashwaghanda, Green Tea and Turmeric in a health supplement. It gave the scientific results of reducing oxidative stress by an average of 40% in 30 days and in 3 months increasing the Glutathione levels by an average of 300%. The amazing thing about this is that the synergy of the natural herbs work so much more effect at helping your body activate the Nrf2 pathway, this is why I recommend this supplement so highly as one of the most effective antioxidants I know off, and as we age the benefits of strengthening your Nrf2 pathway is showing to be one of the most powerful weapons in the fight against aging when it comes to wrinkles and chronic disease. When University of Colorado at Boulder researches gave older mice, aged 70-80 in human years, antioxidant enriched water for four weeks, their arterial regressed to as young as 25 to 35 human years. This Heart health study shows our need for antioxidants becomes more critical as we age. As we age we are more inundated with free radical damage, and antioxidants help neutralise repair this damage.

Our suggestions to you this week:

1. For general health, consider adding in a daily plant-based Mineral complex. Or for a specific health issue please follow the guidelines from your mineral test. To help create a mineral optimization balance in your body

2. Consider adding in a B-Complex if needed or increase your intake of foods rich in vitamin B.

3. Consider adding in a Vitamin D3 & K2 supplement, or make Sure you get twenty minutes of sunshine a day, or use a vitamin D lamp.

4. Consider adding in a omega 3 oil such as one from Cod Liver Oil, Krill Oil & Astaxanthin or Hemp Oil.

5. Consider adding in the Antioxidant Nrf2 Protandim supplement; please go to our website for more information or to order http://yourgreatestwealth.lifevantage.com/.

6. There is a great movie to watch on vitamins called That Vitamin Movie. You can watch it at https://thatvitaminmovie.com/

If you're interested in finding out what are the best health supplements we have come across, on our website we have a page called health supplements which lists of the best and most effective health supplements we have come across.

www.YourGreatestWealth.co.uk

Nature's Remedies

HAVE YOU EVER BEEN IN a health food shop and felt completely overwhelmed by what looks like literally hundreds of different supplement bottles? To add to your confusion, the supplement companies are regulated, meaning they are very limited in what they can say about what their supplements can do for you.

In this chapter we are going to look at five common health issues and which natural remedies can help.

What you soon realise is there is a common theme with helping treat most health conditions, which you simply need to slightly adjust to the condition and the person. Amongst the five conditions are suggestions to help you improve the quality of your sleep (something that will pretty much help anyone). Often joint issues come down to autoimmune disease, so we have a section on that. We'll also look at skin tone, not just from a point of beauty, but using your skin as an indication of your overall health.

The five natural health remedies we will look at are:

1. Improving your skin tone
2. Treating a common cold
3. Healthy heart function
4. Getting the best night's sleep ever
5. Improving joint issues.

Please note: before acting on any suggestion we make here, check with your doctor first that it is compatible with any medication you are already on.

1. IMPROVING YOUR SKIN TONE

Your skin tone is a good indicator of your internal health and there is certain knowledge that can help reduce wrinkles and make you look and feel younger from the inside out.

It comes down to something called oxidative stress, which means that your skin is bombarded by oxidation in daily life, just as an apple that is cut in half goes brown.

The secret is knowing how to reduce oxidative stress or, to put it more simply, to slow down the aging process. The answer is to have an abundance of antioxidants in your body, which helps deal with free radicals, the cause of oxidative stress. Antioxidants act as cleaning ladies to free radicals. You can imagine if the cleaning ladies don't do the cleaning for a few weeks—the rubbish builds up and if this process isn't dealt with, this can accelerate the aging process. Oxidative stress is what toughens the skin and causes wrinkles to appear.

One of the best all-round antioxidants that works on water molecules and fat molecules in your body, and in turn on your skin, is a health supplement called ALA (Alpha–Lipoic Acid). It can actually work like a natural face lift—many people see the benefits of using this supplement within 6 weeks.

You could also add a supplement called Hydrolysed Collagen, which can increase your skin's elasticity, as well as following all the basics such as keeping hydrated, avoiding burnt food and reducing or avoiding refined sugar.

In addition to oxidative stress, the damage to your skin caused by smoking is well documented. If you are a smoker and would like to be totally free of it within 2 hours for the rest of your life, please download Jason Vale's "Stop Smoking in 2 Hours" free app. Jason's app has worked for thousands of people.

Of course quitting smoking also reduces the stress on your heart and reduces inflammation in your body. As you will see in this book, you help one part of your body and it naturally helps other parts. In essence, every chapter in this book can help you to look younger and feel healthier.

2. TREATING A COMMON COLD

Many of our clients report that by following many of the guidelines in this book they have far fewer colds, if any. But if you do have a cold and would like to treat it naturally, here is a suggestion.

Many people turn to antibiotics when they have a cold. The downside of antibiotics is that they are overused and over-prescribed and many bacteria are becoming antibiotic resistant as a result. Antibiotics also kill the good bacteria as well as the bad and can weaken the immune system afterwards (a huge part of your immune system is your friendly bacteria.)

In contrast, the substance Allicin, found in garlic, has been proven for thousands of years to help fight infections without killing the good bacteria. It has been shown to help fight off streptococcus, e-coli, salmonella and many other different types of infections.

Additionally, andrographis is the active ingredient of a Chinese herb called chuan xin lian, known for clearing heat from the body and commonly used for treating infections in the lungs, urinary tract and throat.

The steps for helping treat a common cold:

- Take a high dose of Allicin Garlic and an Andrographis supplement. Follow the instructions on the label and add a natural vitamin C supplement such as acerola cherry, a vitamin D3 supplement and a zinc supplement.

- Sleep and rest as much you can for two days: if you push your body it can take twice as long to clear the cold.

- Avoid junk food, refined sugar and processed foods and eat wholesome, nourishing foods like chicken stock soup and keep the quantity of food down to the minimum for the two days so your body can rest and heal.

3. HEALTHY HEART FUNCTION

Cholesterol is widely considered to be a contributing cause of heart disease. 80% of the cholesterol in your body is made by your liver and the remaining 20% comes from your diet.

If your triglycerides, which supply your body with cholesterol, are high, it means you're eating too many refined carbohydrates, because it's actually sugar that causes triglycerides to rise, not dietary fat.

Just as your diet contains healthy body fat and unhealthy body fat (or put another way, fat that protects your health and fat that promotes disease; the key difference is the presence or absence of insulin sensitivity), there are also both 'good' and 'bad' forms of cholesterol. Contrary to most people's belief, cholesterol is crucial for optimal health as your brain is made from cholesterol and water, and cholesterol is the precursor to hormone production.

A three-year study in Italy measured cholesterol levels in 3000 elderly people. The study found that those with a lower reading (189mg/dl) had a higher risk of death than those with a reading between 276 to 417mg/dl.

When you use drugs like statins to lower your cholesterol, it targets the good and bad cholesterol. A reduction in good cholesterol will lower your testosterone, your muscle tone and can dumb down your brain. The effectiveness of statins is becoming questionable today.

What can help the heart naturally is reducing homocysteine, a natural by-product of your body's metabolism.

If your body cannot break down homocysteine it can have a negative effect on your vascular system by hardening the arteries. Both the British and American medical associations support the use of folic acid, which helps breaks down homocysteine. Brewer's Yeast is the most natural and best form in which to take it.

A hawthorn supplement can also help reduce high blood pressure. Hawthorn contains flavonoids, which help relax arteries and can normalise heart rhythms and chest pains.

With a hawthorn supplement you may not get results overnight, yet most people notice improvements within six weeks. The best time to take hawthorn is on an empty stomach before you sleep. As it helps relax your muscles and increases oxygen intake you sleep better, too.

Several clinical trials have shown that L-Carnitine can be used alongside conventional angina treatments to reduce the need for medicine and improve the ability of those with angina to exercise without chest pain or discomfort. Some studies have determined that taking L-Carnitine after a heart attack decreases the chances of suffering another one later. L-Carnitine helps protect the brain from both age-related and stress-related damage, helping it function longer and better. It also helps reduce body fat, increase muscle tone and increase your energy levels.

4. GET THE BEST NIGHT'S SLEEP EVER

A large portion of your life is spent sleeping, so making this time beneficial makes your waking time the best it can be.

A century ago, the national average was nine to ten hours' sleep; today it is less than seven hours, with the mantra "work harder, sleep less". If you don't sleep well, it doesn't matter what great health habits you have. You're more than likely to be grumpy and it has a knock-on effect on your whole health, from your immune system to your hormonal balance. During waking hours, all your cells get damaged; when you sleep your body repairs your cells and regulates your hormones. Your biological clock controls the rise and fall of the hormones that tell you if you're sleepy or awake and normally most people have two 'energy dips' where they feel sleepy during the day—one after lunch and one after dinner.

I would recommended aiming for about seven and a half to eight hours' sleep per day and, if you can, squeeze in a short twenty-minute power nap after lunch. This is one of the best anti-aging antidotes and it also improves your memory, your awareness and your productivity, reduces anxiety and can increase your happiness levels, so it really is a win-win.

Some people find they sleep better with their head towards the north and their feet towards the south: this is because of the magnetic poles. You can have certain plants in your bedroom, such as lavender or jasmine, that give off smells that ease anxiety, helping you sleep well, and plants such as Aloe Vera or Snake Plant take in carbon dioxide and release oxygen during the night. If you wake near to sunrise and see the first morning light then when it comes to the evening your biological clock is more in tune.

Avoid caffeinated drinks in the afternoon such as green tea and coffee as they are stimulants which will keep you awake.

In the evening it is a good idea to have a cut-off point from screen time or work. You can paint your bedroom with an EMF paint that reduces electromagnetic frequency radiation (which means in short it makes the room feel much calmer). Blackout curtains help darken the room and I would recommend the minimum amount of electrical devices in the bedroom at night. Make the atmosphere in your bedroom relaxing (e.g. soft music and soft lighting) and bedtime is a great time to practice some gentle calming yoga postures or somatic movements that relax the body. You could even do a deep yogic relaxation as you fall asleep.

Other things that may help are taking an herbal valerian supplement, a CBD oil supplement, or spraying your pillow with a product called Deep Sleep Pillow Spray by a company called This Works. All of these can help deepen the quality of your sleep, so you wake up feeling really refreshed and ready for the day.

During a study, Dr. Robert Emmons and Michael Mc McCullough asked people with neuromuscular disorders to write a list of things they were grateful for, before they went to sleep. After only three weeks, participants reported enjoying a longer and more refreshing sleep.

Another recent study led by a Professor Didon suggests that a gratitude practice can help you sleep. When your mind is consumed by positive thoughts there's not so much room for negative ones, which tend to keep you awake.

5. IMPROVING JOINT ISSUES

Joint problems are a major health issue affecting a lot of people. 23% of adults in America have arthritis, which is aching pain, stiffness, and swelling in or around the joints, and a further percentage have mild joint issues.

Some studies have suggested that the foods from the nightshade family (including tomatoes, white potatoes, aubergines and peppers as well as tobacco) contain a chemical called solanine that can make the symptoms of arthritis worse. Many people have reported that omitting these foods from their diet makes a huge difference, but no scientific research has been done to confirm this. Some people report it makes no difference, so our advice if you have joint pain is simply to leave these foods out for four weeks and see what you notice.

Steps to help joint issues:

- Supplement with hydrolysed collagen, which has been shown to help rebuild the collagen between the joints.

- Add a vitamin K2 supplement which plays an important role in bone and joint health.

- Add in a turmeric supplement that is high in curcumin—the medical part of Turmeric that is well known for its anti-inflammatory properties.

- Take an omega 3 oil supplement such as krill oil combined with astaxanthin to help reduce inflammation.

- Pure Turpentine oil from pine trees can be applied directly onto the skin near the joint pain, many people find immediate reduction in pain from using this. (Please make sure you find a natural product that the use is for treating joint pain, and test out a small amount on your skin, to check for any adverse reactions) Turpentine oil has been used as a healing remedy for generations to reduce soreness and muscle pains.

- Take a Vitamin D3 supplement, which strengthens your immune system.

- Avoid lectins: we explain the reasons for this in more depth in our training course.

You could add in a series of Hyperbaric Oxygen Therapy sessions, where you take a seat in an oxygen chamber tank that decompresses the air, replicating the conditions of breathing oxygen at a depth of between five to ten metres underwater. As you breathe in oxygen at this depth it is circulated around your blood at a higher rate than at surface level. This can help decrease inflammation in the body, which in turn reduces pain. Cryotherapy therapy can also ease pain. We will go into both these therapies in more detail.

You could also eat homemade fermented vegetables each day, or take a probiotic supplement which will help increase your gut flora and boost your immune system, or add a Boron supplement which is well documented for helping to soothe joint pain.

An MSM (methylsulfonylmethane) supplement can also help with tissue repair. MSM is the most well-known form of a sulphur supplement, yet there is also a natural supplement that is a waste product of making paper called DMSO. This is very similar to MSM and is known as nature's answer to pain and inflammation.

You can get MSM as a food supplement to take with your meals. DMSO either comes in a gel form that you can paint on your skin (avoid rubbing it in as this can slightly irritate the skin for a few minutes). Dr. Jacob created a low-irritation formula containing 60% DMSO with added vitamin E and a natural oil, which is my preferred choice.

The other downside of using DMSO is that it can make you smell somewhat similar to strong garlic, although this is only when you use it. And if you have joint issues, this is a small price to pay for healthier joints!

A qualified nurse or doctor can give a patient with joint issues a DMSO infusion combined in a saline solution. When I had this, I could feel the benefits almost straight away: it almost felt like oil going directly into my joints and it eased off my pain to a great degree.

Your collagen levels start to decrease in your mid twenties by about 1-1.7% each year. Once you reach the age of thirty, the effects of collagen loss become more noticeable. There are twenty-eight different types of collagen in your body, from your skin and eye tissue to your joints. That is why taking a highly absorbable collagen supplement can help your joints keep feeling young.

Often helping treat any health issue is a combination of many different factors. The expertise lies in setting up the best protocol for you and sticking to it for a period of time to see if it is effective and at the same time combining it with the other elements of this book such as eating the right food for you and having a positive mindset.

Replenishing Adult Stem Cells

I'm always interested in looking at universal underlining causes and what can give my clients the best results. There are certain foods and health supplements that can nourish your bone marrow and in turn this can help activate and replenish adult stem cells, which are like the building blocks and engine for renewing organs, tissue growth, joint health, energy levels and more. This is your health at a cellular level.

The decline of your adult stem cells can lead to unrepaired damage in virtually any body part, leading to tissue breakdown, aging and loss of health. Without active, vigorous adult stem cells good health is compromised long-term.

Scientific anti-aging research shows adult stem cell release rates from the bone marrow drop at an astonishing rate as we age.

- At thirty-five years—the stem cell release rate drops by 45%
- At fifty years—the stem cell release rate drops by 50%
- At sixty-five years—the stem cell release rate drops by 90%

This leaves only 10% of adult stem cells circulating in the bloodstream at age ninety, just when we need them the most to fight disease, sickness and just plain 'getting old'!

In the past, stem cell therapy was only for the rich and famous. It was very controversial because the stem cells were harvested from the umbilical cords of aborted foetuses. More recently, doctors have learned how to harvest the stem cells from the patient's own bone marrow. However, both these options are extremely expensive.

Yet now there is a small selection of foods and health supplements that help activate adult stem cells, which are getting very similar positive results to these very expensive treatments.

The list of those foods and health supplements that are showing that they can possible assist with helping in the circulation of adult stem cells are: Blue green algae, fucoidan in Wakame sea weeds, mesenkine from spirulina, blueberries, green tea extract, L-carnosine, resveratrol, bovine colostrums, vitamin D3 and Lactobacillus Fermentum.

So now when you have your blueberries and green tea in the morning sitting in the sunshine, you now have more of a reason to smile, as these foods can possible help strengthen the circulation of your adult stem cells.

The aim of this chapter is to help you see that when you start combining different parts of natural health in a holistic way, natural protocols can be very effective.

Your homework this week,
if you wish:

1. See if you can get the best night's sleep ever by adding in some suggestions from this chapter.

2. If you have any joint issues and you're looking to soothe the pain naturally, please follow some of the steps above.

3. Consider adding in some of those foods or health supplements from the list above that can help possible increase the circulation of your adult stem cells.

"Your body will be around a lot longer
than an expensive handbag. Invest in
your health."

Power Detox

THERE ARE MANY DIFFERENT TYPES of detox, from semi-fasting one day per week (which can help your body produce new stem cells) to having a proper three-week holiday, where the first week you unwind, the second week you recharge and the third you're re-inspired. Yet many people look after their car better than their body, which doesn't even get a yearly service!

In this chapter I will share with you two of the most simple and beneficial Detoxes I know:

1. A Candida Cleanse
2. A Liver & Gall Bladder Flush

WHAT IS CANDIDA?

Candida is an opportunistic fungus a form of yeast that is the cause of Candida related issues such as fatigue, weight gain, joint pain, and gas.

Candida yeast infection can be found in the mouth, intestinal tract and vagina and it may affect the skin, if the immune system is not functioning properly, the Candida infection can migrate to other areas of the body including the blood.

Most people have some level of Candida in their intestines, and usually it coexists in balance with the good and bad bacteria. But a combination of factors can lead to the Candida population to get out of control, establishing fast growing colonies, and starting to dominate your gut.

At this point it can begin to affect your digestion, weaken your immune system, and even damage your intestinal wall, allowing it's toxic by products to escape into your bloodstream and spread throughout your body.

Why does this happen?

Sadly, more and more people suffer from lowered immune systems due to stress, bad diet, abuse of antibiotics or general ill health. This means the immune system is not strong enough and your beneficial gut bacteria (the good guys that keep Candida in check) are weak or not even present.

Then if there is some damage to the intestinal wall, the Candida yeast can enter the blood-stream where it changes into a fungus with a protective shell and feeds on glucose in your blood.

Candida overgrowth can also cause digestive issues and bowel problems. Candida always resides in the gut, so when an overgrowth occurs it usually starts in the digestive tract. Overgrowth often gives rise to a whole range of digestive issues, including diarrhoea or constipation, bloating, upset stomach, intestinal cramps and irritable bowel syndrome—even bad breath that won't seem to go away, no matter what you do.

Obesity can also stem from Candida. Since it constantly feeds on sugars and carbs, including at night when you're not eating, your adrenals have to work extra hard to compensate for a lack of blood sugar. This eventually leads to adrenal fatigue and low energy levels. As the adrenal glands wear down the thyroid gland also starts to perform poorly, leading to decreased temperature regulation, low metabolism, and weight gain.

Here are some of the most common symptoms associated with systemic Candida:

Thrush	Foggy Thinking	Muscle Weakness
Sore Throat	Itching	Alcoholism
Bloating	Acne	Asthma
Gas	Hyperactivity	Chronic Fatigue
Constipation	Sinus Inflammation	Syndrome
Diarrhoea	Irritability	IBS
Earache	Dizziness	PMS
Migraines	Low Sex Drive	Depression
Fatigue	Athlete's Foot	Anxiety Disorders
Vaginitis	Chronic Pain	Arthritis

As well as poor health, you will notice cravings for sugar, alcohol and carbohydrate-rich foods like bread, pasta, rice etc.

The 5 Way approach

In order to deal with Candida successfully, I have found using this five-way approach gets the best results:-

1. Use a chitin enzyme inhibitor
2. Use anti fungal herbs and oils.
3. Increase the good bacteria
4. Follow the Food Factor guidelines
5. Finish with a liver cleanse

What is a chitin enzyme inhibitor?

Research into Candida bio films is relatively new so our understanding of them is still limited and in progress, but this appears to be one of the reasons why so many people are not able to eradicate their Candida yeast overgrowth.

Candida fungus generates a protective cell wall called a chitin layer that acts as a three dimensional protective shield wall, so it can hide from your immune system. The idea is a chitin enzyme inhibitor works on breaking down this protective layer and when this happens, the white blood cells can overcome the Candida fungus more effectively.

Research suggests that the more mature the bio film, the more resistance that develops. The longer you have had Candida, the more time it has had to develop strong bio films.

There are different type's chitin enzyme inhibitors which you can buy in health food stores and on line, much of the evidence that these work is Anecdotal evidence at present, and I believe more scientific evidence needs to be done in this area.

The chitin enzyme inhibitors that show promise in helping break down the bio films are:

LUMBROKINASE are a group of six enzymes which are able to break down the chitin layer of Candida.

NATTOKINASE is a single enzyme, derived from Japanese fermented soy beans, that works to disrupt the chitin layer.

SERRAPEPTASE this enzyme is derived from the silkworm and, just like the other systemic enzymes, is used to help break down the chitin layer.

What are the antifungals and how do they work?

Antifungals work by either killing the fungal cells—for example, by affecting a substance in the cell walls, causing the contents of the fungal cells to leak out and the cells to die—or preventing the fungal cells from growing and reproducing.

The best natural antifungals I know of are:

TURMERIC / CURCUMIN

A Brazilian research team looked at the effectiveness of Curcumin against twenty-three strains of fungi, including Candida. They found that at a fairly low concentration Curcumin was able to completely inhibit the growth of Candida.

When you use turmeric, you might want to consider taking some black pepper and vitamin C at the same time. There is evidence that black pepper and vitamin C increases the bioavailability of the active compounds in turmeric.

CAPRYLIC ACID

Caprylic acid, sometimes known as MCT Oil, is derived from coconut oil and is one of the most effective natural antifungals, and is so easy to add to your daily food.

OREGANO OIL

Oregano oil is one of the most potent natural antifungals against Candida.

GRAPEFRUIT SEED EXTRACT

Studies of grapefruit seed extract have found it to be highly effective against different yeasts and moulds.

PAU D'ARCO TEA

Pau d'Arco Tea helps to gently loosen the bowels, and also has antifungal and immune-stimulating properties.

LACTOFERRIN

Lactoferrin not only has antifungal properties itself but it has also been shown to increase the effect of other antifungals when taken in combination.

ALLICIN

Is the medicinal part of garlic: it is one of the most useful and well-researched supplemental aids in fighting Candida.

For the Prebiotics and Probiotics

Chicory root is also a great prebiotic, so it can help to repopulate your gut with healthy bacteria too. Chicory root coffee is a good option if you are missing that bitter coffee taste.

For your Probiotics, you can make freshly made fermented vegetables, you can make milk Kefir or water Kefir, or take some probiotic supplements: make sure they have at least six different strains.

BENTONITE FIBRE SHAKE

During your cleanse you can have some of these Bentonite shakes that can help physically clean your intestine.

The fibre part gets your digestive system moving and cleans the walls of your gut, while the super-absorbent Bentonite clay sucks up any toxins sitting in your intestines and carries them safely out of your body.

For the fibre component, there are several different options. Psyllium husk is very effective, but can be a little harsh on the intestines for those who suffer from Leaky Gut Syndrome or who have an irritated intestinal membrane. Another good alternative is pure apple fibre.

Once you have made the drink, drink it straight away and then drink another extra large glass of water immediately after.

RECIPE: FIBRE/BENTONITE SHAKE

1 large cup water
1 level tbsp. fibre supplement
1 level tbsp. liquid Bentonite Clay

This detox drink should be taken on an empty stomach, so don't eat anything for an hour before or after you drink it. The easiest time is usually first thing in the morning, in the afternoon, or a couple of hours before bedtime. You can drink this once a day throughout your cleanse.

When the Candida fungus begins to die off (which is a good thing) it results in the production of toxins in the body.

Your body may go through what is known as the Herxheimer Reaction. This is what happens when the toxin production is too fast for your body to handle properly. Your body will eventually detoxify and eliminate these bothersome fungi but you may feel some unpleasant sensations while you go through this process.

Some of the symptoms you may notice include those similar to having flu. These include headaches, stuffy nose and bodily aches and pains. You may also feel some numbness or skin irritation. You may become constipated or suffer from diarrhoea. Some people may even experience fatigue and mental fuzziness.

Nobody reacts to the die-off process the same way but if you do experience these symptoms you should reduce the antifungals, slow the process down, increase your water intake, have a Bentonite shake and rest well. The aim is to do this cleanse slowly and easily with the minimum of any detox symptoms.

So now we need to put the Candida Cleanse together.

1. Keep on top of the Food Factor guidelines for three months until the symptoms have passed.

2. Start with a Chitin enzyme inhibitors of your choice from the list I've given you. This will break down the chitin layer, then follow the course on the label: this usually lasts around forty-five days.

3. Slowly, at the same time that you start your enzyme inhibitor protocol, start introducing some antifungal foods and herbs as well on a low level. Then, once you have finished the chitin enzyme protocol, continue with these anti fungals at a slightly higher level and let them become part of your normal diet.

4. Throughout the whole time keep adding the good bacteria and aim to take them at a separate time to the antifungals to give them the best chance to do their job.

5. This process should take about three months to complete. The aim now, if you're feeling good and your intestine is in good health, is to finish this process off with a liver and gallbladder flush.

THE LIVER AND GALLBLADDER FLUSH

"Cleaning the liver bile ducts is the most powerful procedure that you can do to improve your body's health."
~ **Dr Hulda Clark**

This liver and gallbladder flush is recommended by many naturopath and herbalists around the world as an overall general clean to the liver and gallbladder to help promote wellbeing. I've personally have done this cleanse myself over a fifteen times spread over 15 years, roughly about once a year . The evidence that I can see that it works is that in the morning I can physically see these green soft stones and I physically feel the benefits by the afternoon. Plus I have heard this same report from many clients, and other Naturopaths who use this cleanse.

Yet caution does need to be taken on this, as it is a very strong cleanse, so if you have any doubts at all please make sure a Nutritionist or Naturopath is supervising you to asses that it is suitable for you.

For best results it is advised that you do a liver flush after having done the Candida Cleanse for a minimum of one month. This detox requires you to follow strict instructions for about twenty-four hours.

Three days before you start the liver flush, drink two large glasses of sour apple juice per day. This will help stimulate the production of bile so you will have a good amount of bile in your gallbladder which will help to flush the stones out.

For each day of the liver flush you will need:

- 4 tablespoons of epsom salts
- ½ cup of olive oil
- ⅔ to ¾ cup of grapefruit juice
- 4-8 L- ornithine tablets
- Pint jar with lid

In The Morning

Take four drinking glasses and fill them halfway with clean, warm water. In each glass place one level tablespoon of Epsom salts. Stir and let the Epsom salts crystals dissolve over the course of the day.

Pour half a cup of olive oil into a lidded glass jar and place in the fridge.

It is vital not to have any fat whatsoever during the morning or afternoon, so that the bile is not used and is saved for the flush. Therefore from when you wake up until 2pm eat plain foods such as quinoa or millet porridge, lightly steamed vegetables or baked sweet potatoes but no oil and no butter at all. It is important to eat plenty of these foods in the morning and at lunchtime in order to keep your strength up and drink plenty of warm water to keep hydrated.

In The Afternoon

From 2pm do not eat anything at all. Keep drinking as much warm water as you like.

In The Evening

At 6pm drink one of the glasses of Epsom salts solution. Sip some warm water in between, but not too much. This will cause you to empty your bowels and have a few loose movements.

At 8pm drink another glass of the Epsom salts solution. Sip a little warm water as needed, but not too much. Again this will cause you to empty your bowels and you will have a few loose movements. The idea of this is that it will help open up the bile duct from the gallbladder to the small intestine.

At 9:30pm, pour half a glass of freshly squeezed grapefruit juice into the glass jar of olive oil.

Take this glass jar up to bed and prepare your bed so you can be perfectly comfortable and relaxed. Take a hot water bottle if you wish. Now visit the bathroom for one last time if you need to.

At 10pm shake the glass jar with the grapefruit and olive oil mix and drink. As you drink the mixture, take four to six L-Ornithine tablets (if you generally have trouble sleeping then take up to eight). This helps remove ammonia and toxins from the body and you will need an extra amount of L-Ornithine for this evening. If you don't take L- Ornithine you may have a rough night and not sleep well.

Lie down and make sure you're totally comfortable, that the pillows are at the perfect height and everything is easy. The more you relax and the stiller you are, the more stones will come out. Make sure you lie still and on your back. Most of the stones tend to pass between twenty minutes to two hours after drinking the mixture so use this time wisely by really relaxing and hopefully falling asleep. You may get a feeling you want to do a poo, but this will be the stones passing through—just stay still and relax. You may want to use visualisation techniques and picture the stones coming out or any relaxation techniques such as soft music in the background.

The Next Morning

When you get up in the morning, drink a little water and another glass of the dissolved Epsom salts and go back to bed. From now on you can drink as much water as you like to rehydrate your body and to flush the stones out of the intestines.

Two hours after the first Epsom salts of the morning, drink the last glass of Epsom salts and rest. In this time you will more than likely pass a lot of small green stones.

Congratulations, you have just cleansed your gallbladder.

A couple of hours after passing the gallstones, you can eat again (around 11am). Begin with some light food like a bowl of soup or some fruit and build up slowly. Take the time to relax in the afternoon to nurture your body. By suppertime you should feel recovered; make sure you take some probiotics to replenish your friendly bacteria.

After you've done one flush, the stones which were stacked up behind come forward and so you may need to do two or three flushes to help clear the gallbladder of soft gallbladder stones. Then you can do this detox once a year as ongoing maintenance.

Your Action plan for this week, if you wish:

1. If you have any signs of Candida overgrowth, please follow the instructions from this chapter.

2. If you have never done a liver flush before and you are concerned about it, please ask a local nutritionist to supervise you. If you are going to do a liver/gallbladder flush, please make sure you do a Candida Cleanse beforehand.

"A healthy outside starts from
the inside"

~ **ROBERT URICH**

Inner Wisdom

" As soon as you trust yourself,
you will know how to live."

~ JOHANN WOLFGANG VON GOETHE

ON THE *YOUR GREATEST WEALTH* Health Generator diagram at the start of this book there is an inner circle called Inner Wisdom.

Your inner source of wisdom and calm has an effect on all the other areas of *Your Greatest Wealth*.

This simple yet fundamental understanding will have a profound effect on your health and wellbeing.

It is in this inner space that you can watch your thoughts; it is in this place you can connect to your pure consciousness; it is a place where you can meditate without meditating, because you're naturally doing it when you connect to this pure consciousness in your daily life.

Yet in our busy lives we can easily become disconnected from this awareness.

When you rest in the space within you in your daily life, it touches every moment of your existence with a breathtaking, heartfelt beauty.

Your level of awareness goes up. You see things more clearly; colours are much richer; your communication with others is clearer; and when you listen, you really hear what the other person is trying to say.

As you experience this more in your life, you start to realize that every mind created issue we have stems from our own thinking, making something mean more or less than actual facts. Sometimes we make things sound more brutal than they actually are, e.g. "This is a nightmare," "I'm so depressed": unknowingly we can hypnotise ourselves and condition our lives with a invisible ball and chain weighing us down.

When we are engulfed in a negative state we can lose ourselves, for example we don't "get" angry, we "do" angry, we act in a certain way, our posture is angry, our voice is angry, our mind is churning the details over, dramatising the event. And yes there may be times you need to show some anger, the question is, when you're angry are you engulfed by your anger? The same is true with worry, anxiety, depression etc, we "do" these states.

Alternatively you can learn how to dance with these challenging states. The secret is first to be entertained by the anger, for example to take that step back from it, watch it, maybe make a light hearted remark, maybe appreciate something, and do this within ninety seconds, not one hour later or one day later after gathering loads of stress hormones, cementing that thought process in, but rather to train yourself to dance with this challenging state within ninety seconds.

Because if you let these emotions let rip, they can cripple you.

As you learn to dance with them, it takes a bit of the energy out of them, by making a light hearted remark, by watching them, by simply labelling it as thinking, the end result is always the same: you end up resting in your inner wisdom. So you can think of this chapter as upgrading the home inside you, the place when you can always find your inner peace.

Each of us has this inner wisdom inside ourselves that lets us rest in this inner space, not in the middle of the hurricane mind, but rather in the space within that can watch the hurricane mind. It melts through any mental anguish and will reveal the clarity and then the next right step is presented and then the next right step is presented, in a direction which feels slightly better.

My experience of this space is that it's as fundamental as gravity. This resting space within us is real and present at all times, yet because it is always there we get so familiar with it that we forget about it.

Just as we can watch our thinking we can also listen to our heart, listen to the intuition in our gut and listen to our sexual centre. In this chapter we will bring it all together as it is all the same thing.

The four steps in this chapter to help you rest more in this inner space are:

1. Awaken the inner wisdom of your mind
2. Tap into the inner wisdom in your heart, gut and sexual centre
3. Learn how to activate this intelligence
4. Discover the benefits of this intelligence

The thing is that if we do not rest within this inner space we can get caught up in our mind as it churns over stressful thoughts. Not only can we make ourselves ill by doing this, the outcome will probably be lose-lose for everyone involved.

Did you know there is often an emotional root cause to most diseases? For example, it may start off with experiencing emotions such as anxiety, sadness or anger, and if these emotions last long enough—over weeks or months—it can cause damage to your physical body.

This happens as you tighten up some of your muscles in response to stressful emotions, then your body produces stress hormones, which can have an effect on your nervous system, which in turn could have an effect on an organ.

If you go long enough without dealing with this emotional issue, it can go even deeper into the body, affecting the health of your bones.

Sadly, in some parts of the world people will deliberately stress and torture an animal before it is killed for meat as they think tougher meat is better for you and will make you a tougher person; in reality it is simply cruel. The reason I mention this is the effect of the stress on the animal's muscles. Why be cruel to yourself? Why torture yourself and toughen up your muscles though long-term stress?

This may sound quite obvious to you; you may be asking yourself why people keep repeating the same old stressful dramas when they have this effect.

There are a few reasons. One is we each have this billion-year-old survival mechanism that works on the logic that even if you hate your job, you're depressed, eat a load of crap food and maybe get drunk to get through the evening, at least you survived!

Well done! Let's repeat that again.

The logic goes that if you repeat the same process, you will survive another day. It is driven by the logical left side of your brain. Anything that includes thriving or living your dreams will be highly questionable to the logical side of your brain, which will try to talk you out of taking even the most minimal risk.

There is also another mechanism that can hold you back from the stillness within.

When I heard of a survey done to discover what people hold most dear in their lives I thought the answers would be things like money, health and family, yet these came way down on the list.

What people held most dear was that their opinion was right! For example, if you are having a conversation or discussion with someone, both of you believe you're correct. Of course sometimes you're right, sometimes you're wrong but this mindset is preoccupied not so much with finding what's true as it is with remaining with the same, blinkered view.

Most people live in separate realities and see things from only their point of view. It is a bit like dealing with a teenager, or someone who is drunk: they know everything.

In my family we have a cup in the kitchen that reads, "I'm not arguing, I'm simply saying why I am right" which sums up this mentality perfectly.

So if somebody is so busy focusing on why they are right, even if they were presented with some incredible piece of information that would make the biggest, most amazing difference in their life, they simply would not hear it.

Most people will hear something and translate it into their own reality. Many times this can create conflict. The secret of this understanding is that wherever there is emotional pain, instead of churning it over in your head, which is unable to see things in a different way, you will learn how to rest in this space within you and connect to your innate wisdom. This will give you insights to firstly accept the situation as it is, then move through it with love. I believe anytime you can show love in whatever you're doing, whether it is making a plate of food or listening to a friend, if you can do it with love the benefits are universal.

When you do this you may realize there are no problems; it is just the illusion of the soap opera your mind has created for you. Then the next truth is naturally presented. You still deal with the situation, yet the qualities of grace, gentleness and wisdom come through.

"What if I told you your beliefs don't make you a free thinker? The ability to change your beliefs based on new information does."

You also may realize that everybody is doing the best they can. We can easily judge someone for doing something wrong but how would we know if, had we had the same day or life experiences as that person, we wouldn't do the same things? I believe that as more people get this understanding, it can literally change the world for the better.

"To solve a problem created by one type of thinking, would you agree you need a different type of thinking?"

DIFFERENT SOURCES OF INTELLIGENCE

The Three Parts of Your Mind

One way to understand this concept is firstly to listen to these insights and then experience it for yourself.

The first thing to understand is there are three parts to your mind.

The first part concerns itself with all the logical, straightforward stuff day to day: one plus one is two, following the steps of a recipe in a cookbook, etc. This is nice and straightforward.

The second part of your mind has, let's say, about ninety thousand thoughts running through it every day. They are a blend of good memories, challenging memories, stories and beliefs.

The stumbling block here is that it's self-sustaining. Let's say you have a random thought in your day of an argument you had a few days ago. Your mind turns this thought into a Steven Spielberg special effect film in your head, churning over the details. How could this person do this? Why are they in denial? Why can this person not see it this way? And so it goes—around and around.

The thing is, as it goes round in your head it produces a negative charge of stress hormones that generates even more stress, which then affects your health. Then, what started out as a random thought has now manifested as actual physical pain. You've made this thought into a physical experience, which gives you even more reason to keep the drama going.

It is exhausting even writing about it! Can you now see clearly how your own thought patterns can create pain in your body?

Luckily, we have the third part of our inner wisdom of our mind: the part where you rest within this quiet space where you can watch your thoughts and, if you listen, you can get those "ah-ha!" moments—insights that feel like a slap on the forehead, that simply humble you and cause you to ask yourself the question "why didn't I see that before?" As you ask better questions, you get better anaswers.

It's a bit like when the Hubble telescope points to just one very small spot in the universe for ten days. At first it looks like there is not much there, yet in those ten days thousands of galaxies and millions of stars are slowly revealed.

Or you could compare it to a dirty, greasy frying pan and all your stress is the grease. If you soak it with water and washing up liquid, in time the grease lifts off by itself.

It is in this quiet watching of random thoughts, stepping back and connecting to this part that is doing the quiet watching, that you tap into an intelligence that is beyond your own mind. You start to realize this intelligence is all around us, whether you look at a blade of grass that knows how to grow roots and photosynthesise, or consider the fifteen million chemical reactions happening in our bodies every second.

Can you see that you can choose to let the first and second part of your mind run your life? That's like letting a teenager run a large business rather than having someone of wisdom and experience at the helm. There's nothing wrong with any of these three parts: they are all beneficial and they all work together. The secret is understanding where it all fits in, and in which order.

Meet the Board

If you learn to access this third part of your mind, it will bring clarity and peace into your life. Yet we are going to take it a stage further. You could see this next stage as a room filled with five people in a fancy boardroom, running a large company. Each one of them has separate skills and insights as to how to make this the best company it can be, and there is one person in charge.

These five areas are your mind, your heart, your gut, your sexual centre and the pure consciousness which rests within all of this.

Each of these centres carries a different type of wisdom that contributes to living an extraordinary life.

Have you ever had a feeling that your mind is saying one thing and your heart is saying something else?

Most people's way of dealing with this could be to say that one centre, such as your mind, dominates the others and discredits the intelligence from the other centres.

If you do not listen to your emotions, a whole host of stress-related illness could affect your gut, which is your emotional centre. If you don't listen to your heart it could cause long-term unhappiness. In essence, they all work together and we are going to show you how.

It may be that you suppress one centre, for example your sexual centre. If your mind prevents you from even asking your partner for a certain massage, for example, your sexual centre may take an opportunity if you're on drunk or drugs. Then when the mind is switched off, it may go completely crazy.

If you can make all these centres your best friends they will all work together in your life and you will access a unique insight from each of them.

Access the Space Within

The first skill to enhance is the ability to listen to these centres more clearly. In short, it's about slowing down.

If you can do this, out of nowhere you'll discover this gentle connection to that part of your intelligence that can watch and rest in these different centres in your body.

There are really no techniques, because all techniques in this are distractions. But I'll share with you a few little tricks that I sometimes use and you may find helpful, too.

The first one is relaxing your jaw. If your mouth is closed or slightly open, see if you can consciously relax your jaw just a little. Try it now: close your eyes for a few moments and feel if you can produce a wave of a relaxation response which emanates from relaxing your jaw.

The second trick is achieving peripheral vision. Let's say you're focusing on something, for example you've been trying for ten minutes to thread a piece of cotton through the eye of a needle—can you imagine how you're feeling? Pretty stressed? The opposite way of looking at something is using your peripheral vision which produces a relaxation response. Sure you need both types of vision for different jobs in life, yet feel for yourself the difference in your heart rate when you focus on something intently compared to using a softer gaze. It is simply another way to activate a switch that can help you relax. The old saying is, "take a step back if you're stressed."

The third trick is, if you're sitting or lounging on a chair, spread your toes, hold for a few seconds and feel the relaxation response. Then squeeze your toes in the opposite direction for a few seconds. Your feet can hold a lot of tension and this helps release that tension. If you're tense it is very difficult to access your inner wisdom.

The idea of using simple relaxation tools is not to get caught up in the technique but rather to use it as a way to access the innate intelligence you already have.

You might ask what to do if you need to make a decision and your heart is saying one thing and your mind says something else.

In a democracy you would say the highest percentage wins, but then the part that loses would be unhappy. The secret is asking the part that said "no" what would make it OK to have a "yes, go ahead". Then, when you listen to this part you may get an insight that the other areas did not see. Then, if all centres are agreed, you can get a "hell yes!" which means every part of you is on board. As a rule of thumb, if you get a maybe, take it as a no.

The more you can rest in this space within you, the more you will see and the more you will access your inner wisdom. One of the side effects is that you start to appreciate the ordinary moments in your life even more. By enjoying the small moments—walking in the rain, enjoying a hot shower, laughing with your friends, having a cuddle, swimming in the sea, sharing a delicious meal, admiring a view, feeling the sun against your face, exchanging a smile—many other moments come into full colour, too. When you're depressed you experience the opposite: things may look like the colour has been drained out.

PUT YOUR INNER WISDOM IN CHARGE

Staying connected to your inner wisdom will take self training, but I hope you'll see it's worth it for the many benefits you'll receive. Use these twelve tips as practical hints to help you move from the 'safety' of letting your mind control your life to the many possibilities and deep satisfaction your inner wisdom can open for you:

1. Don't believe all your thoughts and don't take all of them seriously. Thoughts come and go: most of them are just hot air passing by.

2. Don't try to avoid or deny emotions. You get wisdom from the pain and moving through it with love, not around it or under it. It's best you face it with pure consciousness. If you have to stand up for yourself and say something, say it clearly and to the point without emotional baggage and own your own pain. If you're feeling angry about something, say, "I am angry because…", rather than resorting to blame by saying, "you made me feel angry."

3. Understand that all things come and go. If you're feeling depressed, try to recognise it's not part of you: it comes and goes, just like any emotion. When you're OK about being not ok, this is a sign that you're getting it!

4. Do one thing at a time. You can only effectively focus on one thing, so why try to do more?

5. Turn everyday tasks into appreciated moments. Whether you're cooking the dinner, ironing, chatting to a friend or jumping out of a plane with a parachute on, try to fully experience what you are doing.

6. Practice being curious. It is by being interested in each moment that you discover the magic. There's so much to discover, even if you are in an empty room.

7. Get outdoors and embrace the beauty of nature. What is more amazing than climbing a mountain, walking through a majestic forest or swimming in a crystal-clear river, breathing in that fresh air? When you're in nature, feel that breath bringing you inner calm.

8. Enjoy every bite when you eat. Have you ever had an orgasm eating delicious food? If you haven't, you're missing out on something.

9. Slow down when reading and truly take in the information. Have you ever reached the end of a page in a book only to find your mind is completely blank to what you have just read? With awareness, you can pause more between sentences and really absorb what is being written underneath the words.

10. Remain fully present when listening, without trying to judge or control. Imagine listening to someone without butting in constantly and simply holding the space so that person can fully express themselves and you can truly hear them. It is a totally different way to listen.

11. Take mini-breaks every hour or so when working or studying. Your capacity for concentration is about ninety minutes: taking these small breaks will actually make you more efficient. It's like sharpening your axe every ninety minutes as you cut down a tree: it makes it easier and quicker. Don't work with a blunt axe.

12. Laugh at yourself. If you are Mr or Mrs Perfect, people will find chinks in your armour. Be yourself in all your imperfections: allow yourself and others to see your imperfections and laugh at them. You'll find it easier to connect with others this way.

"Tension is who you think you should be, relaxation is who you are"
~ Chinese Proverb

Action steps this week,
if you wish:

As with all the other chapters, I could set you clear action tasks for the week. Yet In the spirit of opening to your inner wisdom, simply discover the quality of doing nothing and you'll start living more.

The most awesome intelligence does not come from this book, or me, or any other person; it flows through you. The only person who can truly give you these insights is you, through your own direct experience.

This week, my invitation to you is to rest in the space within you, and quietly listen to your innate intelligence. See what you can learn yourself from practising this.

This understanding is like the fabric that makes so many other parts of this book come to life, such as listening in when you're using food Energetics or the techniques in these final two chapters, as you'll soon discover.

"I believe all suffering is caused by ignorance. People inflict pain on others in the selfish pursuit of their happiness or satisfaction. Yet true happiness comes from a sense of inner peace and contentment, which in turn must be achieved through the cultivation of altruism, of love and compassion and elimination of ignorance, selfishness and greed."

~ DALAI LAMA XIV

The Power of You

> " I can be changed by what happens to me.
> But I refuse to be reduced by it."
>
> ~ MAYA ANGELOU

HAPPINESS STARTS WITH YOU: IT'S an inside job. It doesn't start with your relationship, nor with your job, your money or your circumstances, but with you! Have you noticed some people are happy most of the time and some people are grumpy most of the time? Would you like to train yourself to smile more, to laugh more? Did you know you don't get angry, you do angry? Let me explain: when ever you're angry, worried, fearful etc. your body posture changes, whenever you're in one of these states notice where your shoulders are, what is the tone of your voice, are you less tense or more tense, do you talk faster or slower, do you see things working or not working?

What often happens in life is that you keep getting the same challenges until you break through.

As you think it, you become it, this is the voodoo curse. What is your body posture and tone of voice to your health and life?

The idea of this is that you don't just gain the knowledge as a three week fad, that this health wisdom becomes part of your natural nervous system.

Yet if you're playing the victim in your life and you don't know how to step out of it, you may feel like you've imprisoned yourself, and you may not realize how to get out of prison, and this chapter covers your escape plan, if you need it.

VICTIM CONSCIOUSNESS

In India, some parents will cripple their own healthy child's leg so they can beg and get an income.

As sad as it is to say that last sentence, looking back on my own life I have sadly played the victim countless times: disempowering myself and others by manipulating a situation and getting a payoff from it. Sometimes I didn't even realise I was doing it. The point is, I sometimes fell into that place where people do not say what they really want to say. I was brought up in England, the land of the stiff upper lip where it is better to bottle things up than have a tantrum and get things out of the way. When communication gets suppressed it ferments on the inside and, if left long enough, will eat away at someone from the inside out.

Victim consciousness is one of the most dangerous things on the planet: it gives people the excuse to use aggressive language and to be physically violent beyond normal reason. Take the Germans for instance. They used the victim consciousness that the Jews were flooding into their country as an excuse that led to the atrocities of the Second World War. The Germans thought they were the original victims!

Although this is a big extreme example, notice if this following drama triangle that I'm going to explain has come up before in your life and has it affected your health?

Let me explain the characters in the dreaded drama triangle and how it works:

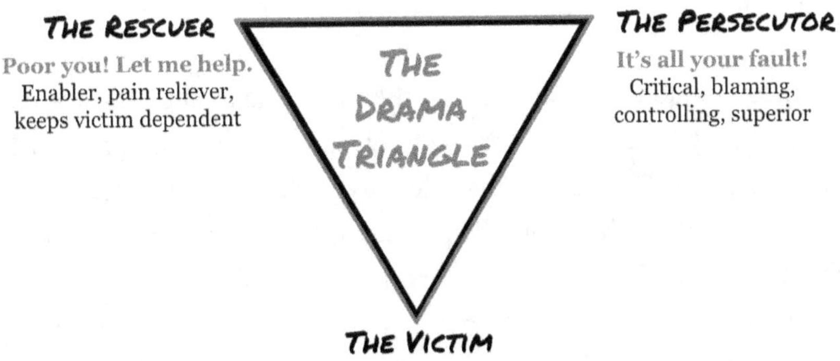

The Persecutor will be putting all the blame on the victim, that it is their entire fault! They will be looking for point scoring. Dominating and controlling most of the conversations. They will have an underlying belief that they are better than the other. They get a pay off being significant and they may act aggressively, be judgemental and will exert their power over others, physically and emotionally. They will fear losing control or being vulnerable which might show they are a victim themselves.

The Victim is preyed upon by the persecutor, the victim will feel helpless and downtrodden, they will complain that their needs are not being met. They will find reasons to avoid self understanding the situation, they will find reasons to avoid making decisions to solve the problem, they will keep busy, juggling many things to avoid getting out of this triangle. The victim will have a deep belief that they cannot solve their own problem, and they get a pay off, of connection or significance from staying in the triangle. They can have a poor me attitude and they think they are without fault or blame. They may take little responsibility in resolving the conflict. They have an underlying belief that the world is out to get them.

Then comes along the Rescuer, for the Victim he or she can save the day and they have a belief that they can sort this out and may attack the persecutor. They are normally are over helpers and pleasers. They may feel guilty if they don't help. They get a pay off, of connection and significance.

They have a need to be needed and to continually give physical and emotional support to the victim.

In turn this will keep the victim dependent on them in a role that can become a burden to them, or lead to accepting the full weight of responsibility for the victim and become a martyr.

So each character is disempowered by each other, it is simply a downward spiral for all three characters.

The danger with these victims' triangles is that the Persecutor then thinks he or she is also a victim of the other two characters, and also finds a rescuer.

The crazy thing in these victim triangles is that everyone is essentially scared of everyone else, and everyone loses in the long run.

The wound is looking to validate its story; the pain wants to be justified; the ego wants to prove it was right. With this mentality you can get caught up in a vicious circle. Luckily, there is a wiser way.

The question that is not asked enough is, "What part did I play in creating the drama triangle if one was created?" Are you feeding the triangle or are you big enough to help melt the corners of the triangle by tapping into your inner wisdom, or finding a coach who can empower you to turn the triangle on its head.

The difference between pain and suffering is that physical pain is just pain, and suffering is a self-inflicted amplification of the pain. A lot of suffering from victim consciousness is self-inflicted.

You might ask why people do this to themselves. Yes, it's because there is a payoff: the ego wants to say it was right. I believe it is also because most people have not been taught how to look at their blind spots or shadows and how to pull back their power from where they once threw it away, not realising the consequence at the time.

Now this leads to the question, how do you pull back your power from a place you don't really want to look at, this blind spot of yours that may be visible to other people, but you would rather not see? This is the journey of becoming a successful shadow hunter.

When you can see your own downfalls and, through looking at them in the way we are about to share with you, you can reclaim your power, it can be uncomfortable and scary for a few moments. Then it is like a celebration.

If you hate your shadows and do not look at them, they will run away or hide and you will more than likely be stuck in groundhog day.

When your mind is churning over something, the skill is to see the wound pattern or victim story in you.

You can ask yourself the question, what is *really* bothering you right now? Or what is it in your life you don't like?

Then be humble. Breathe, be quiet, slow down. Be gentle, because let's face it, looking at your shadows might not be on the top of your to-do list.

Secondly, you need to be smart and patient. Watch the process play out and observe how it makes you feel. Then you might see the part you played in creating the situation, you might see a lesson for you to develop as a person: this is your gift. Even from tough situations, there is often a beautiful insight that you now see with your inner wisdom.

Thirdly, when you can see the part of you that was playing the victim you can either be soft and let your inner wisdom guide you with insights or you can ruthlessly release this stuck energy. You can do this on your own, privately, by having a tantrum like a child, or moving the energy in a wild dance, the point is you move the stuck energy, then your inner wisdom rises to the surface, it is as though the shadow has covered over your inner wisdom and with your expressive movement the shadow fades away.

Some words in the English language contain the letters 'ion'. An ion is a positive or a negative charge. 'Depression', for example, could be seen as pressing down the ions—holding them still, not letting them move. In contrast, 'passion' could be seen as passing the ions—moving stuck ions into passion and energy.

Releasing your shadows is about moving those stuck ions, those charges, in a safe but passionate way. Then, as you slow down from the release, the insights often flood in.

After you have done this exercise you may get insights like, "oh my goodness I was so wrong"; "I didn't see that"; "I can see the other person was doing the best they could from what they knew". These insights are personal to you and only you can discover them in that moment you choose to let them go.

After you've successfully hunted a few of your shadows you may actually look forward to finding more because when you overcome a shadow it feels really great. Because it's in these shadows we find problems that force us to grow; these obstacles are what shape our soul and make us who we are. The problem is people think we shouldn't have problems or shadows so they suppress them or hide them, which is where victim consciousness starts. When you embrace your shadows you will pull back parts of you that you may have lost a long time ago.

Discovering your shadows is a celebration, but you need to be a warrior to do it. Are you a gladiator? Or do your emotions get the better of you? In the on line training I will show you how to do this.

THE MASCULINE AND THE FEMININE

Shadows are sometimes created because people are not taught how to honour their masculine and their feminine energy. You're made up of half of your Mum's and half of your Dad's chromosomes; there are these two special forces that shape our lives, yet very few people really understand them.

So let's go on a journey to understand these two forces a bit more. If we look at the smallest subatomic particles in the universe, what we see are either particles or waves. Particles behave like bullets or a bouncy ball, either penetrating through matter or bouncing back. Waves pass through matter in a wave-like motion. What is interesting is that if you measure these subatomic particles as waves, they will behave like waves and if you measure them as particles they will act like particles. The entire universe—including you—is made up of these subatomic particles.

Let's say particles are masculine energy, and waves are feminine energy. Both have a balancing, beneficial aspect for your life. The true question is, how developed is your inner masculine energy? How developed is your inner feminine energy?

Try asking yourself some questions: how old is your masculine energy—is it a mischievous little boy or a well-rounded, loving mature man? Or how old is your inner feminine—is she a little spoilt girl or a fully embodied woman?

This is not about how much you have of either energy. It is about how well-developed they are and how you develop them in your life. Do you learn from your lessons, or are you stuck in your dramas?

Is one side dominating and bullying the other, which may feel like there is an internal war or conflict inside you?

When you start nourishing the best in both, you feel like a well-matured grand reserve bottle of wine: it's juicy, it's tasty, something to be enjoyed.

The masculine is great for aiming for a goal, holding the space, straightforward action, to be challenged to grow, being efficient. It loves that place of no thinking, or empty awareness, that place where a mission is completed and then there is the satisfaction of emptiness.

Whereas the feminine energy is everything. It loves to been seen, it loves to create. It likes compliments, it likes attention, it's chatting to your neighbour, it's cuddles and kisses, it's watching the sunset.

Yet when the feminine is going around in circles getting confused about being confused, the inner masculine can stay the course. The period of pregnancy is feminine, the point of giving birth is masculine. When the inner masculine pushes towards the goal, hurting itself, the feminine can show the emotional pain.

As you can start to see, both sides are part of the same coin. Both sides are needed: one cannot be without the other. The coin can either be in union or internal conflict.

The cool part of this entire chapter is that there is this deep knowing in you that already knows about this healthy balance, which is why change can happen so quickly.

This may be a bit deep, but there is a beautiful insight if you're ready for it. The essence of your inner masculine side is pure awareness: it's this part of you that is empty of thought. It's the man-cave thing, the place that simply watches what is going on, and when you look at this part of you that is simply reading these words and waiting for the next words you might realize this part of you has never aged or changed and was never born and will never die.

The essence of your inner feminine is creative. A lot of things are going on: there are people to talk to, things to see, which constantly gives birth to new experiences and also brings death to old experiences. This is the constant circle of life and death, so your inner feminine never dies. This shows you there is a part of you that is eternal.

So on a deep level, nothing can really happen to you. Your emotions can get hurt but you're not your emotions. Your essence is love and when you penetrate the world with love you go from having an ordinary life to an extraordinary life.

The opposite of giving yourself stress is giving yourself pleasure. If you know how to do that, whether you're relaxing on a sun bed, combing your fingers through your hair or making amazing love with your partner, it is about loving yourself in a beautiful way.

When you can love yourself in this beautiful way you also become a better lover. If you can truly know your operating system, that is you know which parts of your body get pleasure from being touched in a loving way, then when you meet your partner in this way it is like you're already full. Then in your relationship you're exploring each other's fullness rather than just meeting basic needs.

When you can clearly say to your partner I like this, I don't like this and know how to say no and yes clearly, this indicates to your partner that you know how to look after yourself. They can relax and don't need to be a psychic detective trying to guess what to do. When you see a "NO" as someone taking care of themselves, rather than taking it personally, it's a gift to you both as you no longer need to apologise for you being you. Speaking clearly without any manipulation shows how developed you are and leads to the most beautiful experiences to making love, to loving your life.

> *"Rise above the storm and you will find sunshine"*
> **~ Mario Fernandez**

Suggestions for this week, if you wish:

1. Keep an eye out for any shadows that may come up this week. Become a shadow hunter by following the instructions above.

2. Look at how you can honour your inner masculine and inner feminine and start seeing this energy all around you—from empty shelves with square edges (masculine) to shelves that are full of stuff and have soft, round edges (feminine). See if you can create more union between these two forces in your daily life.

3. Find three or more ways to bring more pleasure to yourself this week.

There are things that are kept secret out of fear and there are things kept secret because they are sacred. In this chapter I can only really share a small amount on this subject because it's so huge.

If you are interested in pulling back your whole power and living fully there is a training course called *ISTA Temple Arts, Level 1* that is run all around the world. It covers some of the things I've mentioned plus much, much, more.

Your Perfect Life

> " Believe you can and
> you're halfway there."
> ~ **THEODORE ROOSEVELT**

YOU MIGHT ASK HOW GOAL setting or living your dreams has anything to do with your health! When you're living at ease with yourself, living with passion and purpose, the feel-good chemicals you get from this have a huge effect on your health.

Too often people with health conditions start to shrink in their dreams. They learn to live with self-esteem issues and feel like they are in a self-made prison. Yes, I understand there may be restrictions, yet there are ways to start living your dreams today and ways to feel truly alive. This chapter gives you some of those tips that will help activate this in you, no matter what your circumstances.

In this chapter you'll discover six key areas that will help you live a life you love. These are:

1. The Happiness Advantage
2. Regrets of the Dying
3. Book-ending Your Day
4. Living the Million Pound Lifestyle, Starting Today
5. Your Six Basic Needs
6. Vision Boarding

THE HAPPINESS ADVANTAGE

A lot of people's lives are about studying at school and university for about fifteen years of their life. They work forty years doing a job they don't really like and then, when they retire, they wonder which will last longer, their money or their health.

The modern day formula for happiness unfortunately sets us up to be unhappy and raises the question of how you can start to love life.

Many companies and schools around the world follow the formula that if you work harder you will be more successful, and if you're more successful you will be happier.

The issue is backward for two reasons: firstly because every time you have success you just change the targets. You have good grades so you start aiming for even better grades. You have a well-paid career, now you must look for an even better-paid career. You hit your sales target then you increase your sales target.

Here is the thing: if happiness is on the other side of success your brain will never get there. We are creating a society that pushes happiness out of reach.

The brain actually works in the opposite way. If you raise positivity in the present, then the brain experiences what is called a happiness advantage, and your brain performs significantly better than in a negative, neutral or stressed state. Your energy levels rise; your creativity rises; you're more resilient and less likely to burn out. You achieve greater sales, a better, more secure job, better grades. You still reach amazing goals but this way it's win-win: you reach your goals and you're happy along the way.

To emphasize this point, in America someone commits suicide every 12.8 minutes. The biggest cause of death between the ages of fifteen and twenty-four is suicide and in a general survey undertaken in America in 2014, 60-80% of people were unhappy with their job. In the UK, 12% of the population are on antidepressants.

Let's get things into perspective. Worldwide, 15% of people are malnourished, 14% don't have the ability to read, only 30% are active users of the internet, 37% lack basic sanitation and 48% live on less than $2 a day. If you can read and write, have access to the internet and you earn more than $2 a day, you are luckier than 80% of the population of the entire world. But if you focus on your lack, that is what you will see. The insight here is to start focusing more on your abundance and on your appreciation.

So what really makes us happy? Harvard University have spent 75 years researching what makes people happy and they found the top reasons for unhappiness are loneliness or (even worse) being in a bad relationship. The top reason for happiness was having a handful of really good friends and a loving family or being in a loving, caring relationship. When people had these things the statistics showed they lived longer, enjoyed their lives more, and were more successful in what they did.

REGRETS OF THE DYING

How can we avoid an unhappy life? One way is to look at the top regrets dying people express and then reverse-engineer them to avoid having the same regrets ourselves. So here are the top things dying people say they regret:

1. I wished hadn't worked so hard on work I didn't enjoy.
2. I wish I'd stayed in touch with my friends.
3. I wish I'd let myself be happier.
4. I wish I had had the courage to express my true self.
5. I wish I hadn't been afraid of others people's opinions and had lived my life true to my dreams instead of what others expected of me.
6. I wish I'd travelled more when I had the chance.
7. I wish I had played more with my kids.

If we look at the list above and decide to turn each statement around, the new list might look something like this:

1. I take control of my life and take full responsibility for the things that happen to me.
2. I limit my bad habits and lead a healthier life.

3. I'm not afraid to do what makes me happy.
4. I feel closer to my friends and family.
5. I understand myself better; I know who I really am.
6. I have a new sense of meaning and purpose.
7. I'm better able to focus on my goals and dreams.

The average life expectancy in the UK is 78.1 years and science has proven that if you're happier your body will live longer.

So if you can find ways to keep happier you will live longer, it is scientifically proven.

BOOK-ENDING YOUR DAY

"Light Tomorrow with Today"

~ Elizabeth Browning

There are many ways to start and end your day well: as you can guess it has a great effect on your day. If you can prime your state at the beginning and end of your day this will have a massive impact on your health.

There are many ways to do this and I will show you in the video course. One suggestion is when you wake up tomorrow morning shout, "YES, YES, YES!" and punch your arm up in the air as you do it. You might think it's crazy, yet it's far more crazy waking up with thoughts like, "I hate my life; I feel crap; I don't want to go to work" or running the previous day's argument over in your mind. Instead, you're smiling and your state will be in line with success.

I recommend you avoid turning on social media first thing. Instead, keep this first period of the day for you: maybe meditate for ten minutes using an app like Headspace, go for a run or do something like tai chi, dancing, yoga or whatever kind of exercise you like. The first part often sets the energy for your day.

If you don't like waking up in the morning and embracing your day, it's time to have a good look at the structure of your life. Everything is showing you something.

A morning meditation is also another great way to start your day. Here is a short and powerful meditation for you to try:

Firstly, light a candle. Take a moment to close your eyes and set aside ten minutes to enjoy this exercise to align your state with your day.

To begin, think of what you are grateful for in this moment—it may be the smallest of things or the biggest—or remember a moment from the day before you are grateful for and let your gratitude flow naturally for about three minutes. Let your creativity be engaged so it feels authentic and powerful.

For the second stage, think of something that might be a slight challenge for you in your life, and give thanks for this. Again, engage your creativity; let it feel authentic and powerful. Take about two minutes on this.

Thirdly, take a moment and give thanks for your inner wisdom. Tap into your inner wisdom and rest in this place where you can simply watch your thoughts.

Then if you wish, you can use your imagination to visualise your day. See what you're going to achieve today, how you're going to be. Again, let your creativity be engaged in it so it feels authentic and powerful. Do this for about five minutes.

The secret to doing things like this, or going to the gym, is that you celebrate afterwards, you say to yourself that was awesome, so it becomes your default setting, it gets into your nervous system, so you crave it. Then you say to yourself this is how I rock!

Then whatever you do is at an outstanding level, it maybe only be 2mm more from plain good, yet that 2mm of going that extra bit further gives you that growth , which is one of your basic needs, then you really feel alive, live your life to the full, it is only by raising your standards that your life changes. And you either do this by moving away from massive pain or moving towards pleasure.

What can stop you is FEAR and you can choose what it means.

Fuck Everything and Run or Face Everything and Recover. What do you choose?

As you change your internal emotional environment you in turn change your outside environment and very soon you see incredible things happening in your life that you can't even imagine right now.

LIVING THE MILLION POUND LIFESTYLE, STARTING TODAY

The first trick is to start living your success—now! It's not about the million pounds in the bank, it's about having a million-pound lifestyle which has freedom in it. The important fact is you can start living the millionaire's lifestyle today without the million pounds in the bank.

Be creative with what resources you have. Start hanging out with people who are already successful in the field you love; have luxury holidays in places that are cheap to travel; join a classy gym if you wish. See what ideas you come up with when you think outside the box.

As you start hanging out with successful people in the field you love, you are much more likely to get and see more opportunities to live your dreams.

I always carry about £300 in my wallet. It's not that I spend it carelessly, I do it to feel abundant and it's this feeling that makes the difference. If you like, try it for yourself and see if you notice any difference in your mental and emotional state.

Unsuccessful people see things as they are and then imagine the worst outcome; successful people see things as they are and envision a great possible outcome come true. Your imagination is like the prelude to what comes next in your life. Your imagination is the key to your dreams.

If you don't design your own life plan, chances are you'll fall into someone else's plan and guess what? They probably haven't got much planned for you. Ask yourself when was the last time you upgraded your phone, then when was the last time you upgraded your life? Think about what poor people read and don't read it, what poor people watch on television and watch something else.

YOUR SIX BASIC NEEDS

In life we have six basic needs and these come into play into every area of your life, from your relationships, your business, literally everything. The six basic needs are:

1. You need certainty. This is about your survival mechanism. For example, you have a place to sleep, you have food and you have a job.
2. You need uncertainty. If everything is too much the same it's boring: you can't think or see outside the box.
3. You need to grow. Enjoy the fun of learning and exploring new skills.
4. You need to be significant, so there is something you shine at in life.
5. You need to give and receive love and connection (how are your relationships?).
6. You need to contribute, to give beyond yourself, to care for and serve others.

The thing to ponder on now for five minutes is: looking at these six basic needs which ones are neglected in your life? Which ones are the strongest? Which needs are lacking in your business? Which needs are lacking in your relationships? What I realized is if significance is at the top, there is always going to be someone better than you at what you do, so then you may feel unsatisfied most of the time. Yet if growth, contribution and love were at the top there are no down sides to basic needs, so the question is, is it worth changing some priorities around?

Whatever good or challenging situation you're in, in life these six basic needs will be playing a fundamental role, and if you have at least three of them in the positive you will be addicted to that situation. If you don't have any of them you will have no passion towards it.

> *"If I am only happy for myself, many fewer chances for happiness. If I am happy when good things happen to other people, billions more chances to be happy!"*
> **~ Dalai Lama XIV**

Once you start asking better questions, you will get better answers. One good question to ask yourself is what's your purpose? Or putting it another way, how do you show you're significant in the world?

The two most important days of your life are the day you're born and the day you find your purpose, your passion, and start fully living from your heart.

> *"Your Purpose is to find your Purpose"*

Instead of asking yourself what the world needs, ask yourself what makes YOU come alive, and then do THAT, because that is what the world needs—people who have COME ALIVE.

"I hope everybody could get rich and famous and will have every-thing they ever dreamed of, so they will know that it's not the answer."
~ Jim Carey

There isn't anything wrong with material things, the point Jim is making here is to feel happy even if you don't have the trappings of material things. It's as much about the journey and experience as the end destination. So you can have the best of both worlds as long as you're not just obsessed with material things or turn into a flaky hippy with no drive or passion at all.

You can find a balance between being driven toward your dreams and feeling completely fulfilled in this moment as you are. They may seem like opposite forces, but they complement each other.

If I ask you the question what is it you would most like to create or have happen in your life, what would it be?

Many people's answers are things like a new car, a loving relationship, a bigger home, more holidays, better health and so on.

This is all great, but there is an illusion here. It's not so much about the things people think they're looking for, it's much more about how those things make them feel.

The goal is to experience on a daily basis the feeling of driving away the new car from the garage, being in that loving relationship, starting that new diet. You can of course get these things, but after a time that feeling or motivation wears off and you decide to chase another thing, another diet or another relationship to drive away the emptiness.

The thing with chasing things is that they're always out of reach. If you're chasing money and things with money is it is a number. The thing with numbers is they go on to infinity; there is no end. Your desire can never be fulfilled so you're left with an emptiness which is always hungry for more.

VISION BOARDING WITH LASER-LIKE VISIONING

We now come to the magical technique that will bring your dreams into reality, which is how to create a vision board that really works.

You may think you've heard everything there is to know about vision boards and, because of the law of familiarity, you may discard any possibility of value. Or maybe this is your first time creating a vision board which is fantastic because when you look at something with fresh eyes, you often get the best results. As I've been teaching this for a long time now you are going to get the latest insights to make this super powerful.

Without a vision for our goals we can easily get lost. You could compare it to programming your sat-nav. Have you ever set off on a journey without programming your sat-nav and got really lost? Did you wish you'd taken the time to programme it before you left? Well, putting some pictures on your vision board is like setting your sat-nav to your destination.

The basic idea for your vision board is to find a large cork pin board or a large sheet of paper where you can glue or pin a collage of pictures that represent some of your dreams and aspirations.

Many people make the mistake of putting on too many unrealistic, abstract pictures that are not aligned with what is really in their heart.

The secret to making a truly amazing vision board for yourself is integrating the information that resonates with your inner wisdom. Then you can find images on Google Images, Pinterest, Instagram, or in magazines. The first picture should be a vibrant picture of you. If you have a partner or family, choose a group picture and place it in the middle.

Then brainstorm questions like what is really important to you, what pictures come to your mind? Looking at the six basic needs list from above, ask yourself which of these need some attention in your life and see what images come to mind. Do you have a business plan? If you do, include a picture that shows a clear target for your business.

You may also like to imagine the amazing holidays you'd like to go on, your dream home, a health retreat holiday you would like to attend. Anything that comes to your mind, consider it and then choose the best of the best images for that. If you make it wishy washy, without investing any energy into your choices, the results will be poor. Yet if you turn the dial inside you to give it laser-like focused energy you'll find you get outstanding results.

I used to instruct people to divide their vision board into certain areas. Although this works, I have found that sometimes the less instruction you receive and the more creative you are with your vision board, the more you make it your own and really use your inner wisdom to work out the best pictures. This results in an extraordinary vision board.

On my board, one of my pictures is an image of Usain Bolt winning a race with a caption above it saying this is how I'll feel when I finish my book. I've also added a completion date: there is a forfeit for me if I don't complete it and there is a reward for me if I do. The point is, it points to a feeling. This is a clue: if a picture on your vision board gives you a feeling that feels like a YES, this feeling is one of the main secret ingredients to a laser-like vision board.

Remember reasons come first; answers come second. When you can look at your board and get goosebumps, feel motivated and excited about it, the energy of this feeling makes things happen.

"No matter what happens in your life stay faithful to your dreams"

When you talk about your vision it is a dream! When you plan you make it possible! And when you take action you make it happen.

Whatever you want to specialise in, immerse yourself in that environment, with the best people in the world in that area, then go away, practice it and then go back again to make those final tweaks, then get out into the world and share your passion at an outstanding level. Because mediocre or good does not cut it anymore, before the financial crash in 2008 maybe you could get away with good, but not any more.

Monthly Candle Vision

You're coming to the end of this book and this is the final technique to help you activate your vision board.

Step one: buy a really nice good quality candle. On the first of each month, light the candle and follow the next two steps.

Step two: look at your vision board and ask yourself the question. "What baby steps or giant steps can I make happen or achieve this coming month?" Write the answers down on a piece of paper and stick it on your calendar.

Step three: close your eyes and picture in your mind's eye those steps being achieved. Have a sense of reverence and use as many senses as you can. Try to feel, hear, see, smell and taste the experience. Try to sense some movement—if you truly engage the senses of seeing, hearing, feeling, and some movement this is where you can affect your paradigm. Have some music on in the background.

This short ceremony may last only last roughly nine minutes, once a month; the important thing is the quality of what you feel in your whole body as you do it. When you're done, simply blow the candle out knowing that you have aligned yourself to your dreams and sent your wishes out to the coming month.

Now each day you can start to chunk down your vision into smaller, manageable steps for that day, you can make a "to-do list", then reduce that to a "must-do list", leaving only what is most important. Once you have this, you have a clear focus for each day. Also, do the hardest task first, then the rest is easy.

Your daily goals will change. Sometimes your goal could be to have fewer goals and more free time; it could be simply managing your work-play balance; it could be to be more relaxed. Whatever it is, you can shape your life how you like—your life is literally in your hands.

By taking these action steps and creating healthy habits you are back in control and ready to self-actualize your life.

> *"If you love life don't waste your time for that is what life is made from"*
> ~ **Bruce Lee**

Your practical action steps for this week, if you wish:

1. What motivates you to live your dreams? Write three reasons in each of these areas of massive pleasure you will gain when you achieve this in your: Physical Health, Emotional States, Relationships, Time Management, Career/Mission, Finances and how you celebrate and enjoy your life and then do three reasons in each of these categories on the massive pain you will feel if you don't achieve it.

2. Out of the regrets of the dying which are the two that most resonate with you? When you reverse that list, which two would you like to add more of in your life?

3. Experiment with trying the three cries of "YES!" tomorrow morning and test out the morning mediation. Notice the effect it has on your day.

4. How can you live more of your dream lifestyle, starting today? List three things you can do this week that tell you you're living that lifestyle already.

5. Get 30% of your vision board completed this week!

The key insight in this chapter is about your paradigm. This is your vibration, your state: it is knowing that your dreams are often on the other side of your comfort zone and having the ability to step up, to make your move. It's your posture; it's your internal self-talk; it's how you wake up in the morning, it is how you go to sleep. Your paradigm is asking yourself questions like, "What is the most fun thing I can do today? How do I rock?"

Because this moment is your miracle: your life is your greatest gift, if you can appreciate a smile you're wealthy. This is your abundance frequency.

"Never give up, for that is just the place and time that the tide will turn. Life always gives you a second chance and it's called tomorrow."

Conclusion

AS YOU CAN NOW SEE, your Greatest Wealth is merging together many different investments in your health, from reducing your toxins to drinking yourself healthy; from eating yourself healthy for you to supporting your body with essential supplements; from using natural remedies to having a power detox cleanse. It's resting in the space within, with your inner wisdom, becoming a shadow hunter, living your dreams, laughing more, dancing more, smiling more and seeing how all these different areas come together.

My wish for you is that you try some of these suggestions that I've learnt from many great teachers and discover what really works for you. Make it your own so your discover your greatest wealth.

As your Greatest Wealth is your health, the greatest wealth for our planet and our next generation is our environment. So making more eco-friendly choices that also benefit our health is our greatest wealth of all.

"On a daily basis the greatest gift you can give to yourself is your happiness and health"

Be Well, Be Happy, Be Healthy, Be Awesome
Tony Be

Endnotes

Introduction

1. 2011/2012 Survey National Statistics NHS On Obesity Physical Activity and Diet.

2. It is now predicted that children today are expected to live ten years less than their parents: this is the first time in history a paper published in the New England Journal of Medicine predicts a decrease in life expectancy due to obesity rates.

3. Lesley M.Russell. "Reducing Disparities in Life Expectancy: What Factors Matters?" A background paper prepared for the workshop on reducing disparities in life expectancy held by the roundtable on the promotion of health equity and the elimination of health disparities of the Institute of Medicine, February 2011

4. J.Lazarou, B.Pomeranz, and P.Corey. "Incidence of adverse drug reactions in hospitalized patients." Journal of the American Medical association 1998

5. Michelle Chen. "Discovery of toxins in newborn blood causes alarm." New Standard July 21 2005

6. Are Your Toiletries Toxic Mail Online july 2009

Cleanse Balance and Align

1. B.Jackson "Cosmetic consideration and nonlaser cosmetic procedures in ethnic skin." Dermatologic Clinics 2003

Liquid Health

1. Environmental Working Group. "A national assessment of tap water quality." (More than 140 contaminants with no enforceable safety limits found in the nations drinking water.) 20 December 2005

2. National Research Council. Fluoride in Drinking Water: A Scientific Review of EPA's Standards. Washington, D.C The National Academies Press 2006

Food for Life

1. The Adventist Health Study 2014 Concluded vegetarian diets associated with an overall lower incidence of colorectal cancer World Cancer Research Colorectal Cancer Statistics 2012

2. The oil guide: which to use for frying, drizzling and roasting The Telegraph 10 November 2015

3. Which oils are best to cook with BBC On Trust Me, I'm a Doctor July 2015

4. Linus Pauling Mineral Defiency, Micronutrient Information centre Oregon State University

Power Supplements

1. Harris Gardner "Study finds supplements contain contaminates. " New York Times 25 May 2010

2. William Cromie "B vitamins cut heart disease risk for women." The Harvard University Gazette February 1998

3. Ann Walker, et al. Omega 6 Oil and harmful effects Corn Oil in Treatment of Ischaemic Heart Disease 1965

4. Increasing homicide rates and linoleic acid consumption among five Western countries, 1961-2000. Us National Library Of medicine, National Institutes of Health

5. Evolutionary aspects of diet, the omega-6/omega-3 ratio and genetic variation: nutritional implications for chronic diseases 2006

6. N-3 polyunsaturated fatty acids in coronary heart disease: a meta-analysis of randomized controlled trials The American Journal of Medicine

7. F.J. Giblin. "Glutathione: a vital lens antioxidant." Journal of Ocular Pharmacology and Therapeutics 2000

8. "Sunshine might stop skin cancer" BBC News February 2005

Natural Remedies

1. Lester Packer , Eric Witt, and Hans Jurgen Tritschler. "Alpha Lipoic acid as a biological antioxidant." Free Radical Biology and Medcine 1995

2. Anna Bilska and Lidia Wlodek . "Lipoic acid—The drug of the future?" Pharmacological Reports 2005

3. Sirakarnt Dhitavat, "Acetyl-l-Carnitine protects against amyloid-beta neurotoxicity: Roles of oxidative buffering and ATP levels."Neurochemical Research 1990

4. A.Pares, et al. "Effects of Milk Thistle (Silymarin) in alcoholic patients with cirrhosis of the liver :results of a controlled, double-blind, randomized trial."Journal of Hepatology

5. E.H. Reynolds. "Folic acid, aging, depression, and dementia." British Medical Journal 2002

6. Avery Johnson. "A risk in cholesterol drugs is detected, but is it real?" Wall Street Journal

7. ILSA Group "Low total cholesterol and increased risk of dying: Are low levels clinical warning signs in the elderly?" (Results from the Italian Longitudinal Study on Aging.) Journal of the American Geriatrics Society 2003

8. K.M. Anderson, W.P. Castelli, and D.Levy. "Cholesterol and Mortality." (Thirty years of follow-up from the Framingham study.) Journal of the American Medical Association 1987

9. Naveed Akhtar. "Is homocysteine a risk factor for atherothrombotic cardio-vascular disease?" Journal of the American College of Cardiology 2007

10. Anti-Bacterial Effect of Garlic against Staphylococcus and E Coli Journal of Infectious Diseases November 2016

11. Do Statins Produce Neurological Effects? Scientific American

12. Lancet Study on statins was fundamentally flawed The Telegraph November 2016

13. How a collagen pill can beat arthritis Daily Mail

14. The essential oil of turpentine and its major volatile fraction Research Gate January 2009 Pub Med

Power Detox

1. Curcumin as a promising antifungal of clinical interest Journal of Antimicrobial Chemotherapy 1 February 2009,

2. Coconut oil can control overgrowth of a fungal pathogen in GI tract; study in mice suggests Science Daily November 2015

www.ingramcontent.com/pod-product-compliance
Lightning Source LLC
Chambersburg PA
CBHW050815260726
48660CB00004B/1435